The Woman's Guide to Managing Migraine

The Woman's Guide to Managing Migraine

Understanding the
Hormone Connection to
find Hope and Wellness

SUSAN HUTCHINSON, MD

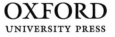

OXFORD
UNIVERSITY PRESS

Oxford University Press is a department of the University of Oxford.
It furthers the University's objective of excellence in research, scholarship,
and education by publishing worldwide.

Oxford   New York
Auckland   Cape Town   Dar es Salaam   Hong Kong   Karachi
Kuala Lumpur   Madrid   Melbourne   Mexico City   Nairobi
New Delhi   Shanghai   Taipei   Toronto

With offices in
Argentina   Austria   Brazil   Chile   Czech Republic   France   Greece
Guatemala   Hungary   Italy   Japan   Poland   Portugal   Singapore
South Korea   Switzerland   Thailand   Turkey   Ukraine   Vietnam

Oxford is a registered trademark of Oxford University Press in the UK
and certain other countries.

Published in the United States of America by
Oxford University Press
198 Madison Avenue, New York, NY 10016

© Oxford University Press 2013

Library of Congress Cataloging-in-Publication Data
Hutchinson, Susan, 1956–
  The woman's guide to managing migraine / Susan Hutchinson.
  pages cm
  Includes bibliographical references and index.
  ISBN 978-0-19-974480-0 1. Migraine—Treatment.   2. Women—Health
and hygiene.   3. Self-care, Health.   I. Title.   II. Title: Guide to managing migraine.
  RC392.H88 2013
  616.8'4912—dc23
  2012037067

Conflict of Interest/Disclosure Statement:

Susan Hutchinson, MD, is on the Speakers Bureau for Allergan, Forest, Impax, and Zogenix.
She has served on Advisory Boards for Allergan, Forest, MAP, NuPathe, and Zogenix. She is
not employed by any pharmaceutical company nor does she own stock in any pharmaceutical
company. She has not received grant money from any pharmaceutical company.

9 8 7 6 5 4 3 2 1
Printed in the United States of America
on acid-free paper

Contents

Preface

Why write a book on women, hormones, and headache? Aren't migraines easy to manage? The short answer is that it is my passion to help meet the needs of the more than 22 million women in the United States who suffer from migraine headache. Headache in women is a major health issue and one that deserves special attention. Too many women are suffering from disabling headaches, mainly owing to improper diagnosis and inadequate treatment. My goal for this book is to help women with headaches get the right diagnosis and get on a treatment plan that will give them the quality of life they deserve.

Many self-help headache books are available in the health and medicine section of bookstores, yet none is devoted specifically to women, with a focus on hormonal factors and how they relate to women's headaches. (Interestingly, the women's health and medicine section of a large bookstore I visited recently was filled with hormonal advice for women dealing with menopause and perimenopause, as well as a myriad of other women's health issues, but there were only a small handful of books in the headache section.)

I saw a new patient this past week in my practice. Tearfully, she told of her kids' drawings showing her lying in bed. She has missed countless school performances owing to her disabling migraines. She spends many vacation days staying in their hotel room while her husband and kids explore. Is this the memory that her kids will have of their mother?

I want to give this patient her life back, to be fully engaged with her husband and kids, and to live her life despite her headaches. Too many women with headache live their lives "around" their headaches, tip-toeing through life, afraid of all possible triggers that can disrupt their days. I cannot cure migraines, but I can help women in my practice find effective treatment and get back to living the lives they deserve—as free of disabling migraines as possible.

Who am I? I am a family medicine physician with a specialty in headache. I also suffer from headaches. Countless women have told me their headache stories over my past 30 years of practice. I have become the headache doctor I am today because of the trust my patients have put in me, the patience they have demonstrated when initial treatment regimens fail or bring unwanted side effects, and their commitment to working together in partnership with me to do everything we can to minimize the impact of headaches on their life.

The field of headache medicine has witnessed incredible advances in recent years. My goal is to help explain to you, the headache sufferer, what we know. I want to empower you to understand as much as you can about your headaches. Understanding the relationship between hormones and headache is critical for women headache sufferers. Traditionally, neurologists have been the specialists that patients with headache are referred to by their primary care physicians. However, in general, neurologists don't understand the relationship between hormones and headache. They don't conduct well-woman exams and make decisions about birth control pills and hormones, as I have over the course of my career. In contrast, gynecologists are very comfortable with making decisions about hormonal treatments for birth control or menopausal symptoms but are often uncomfortable with headache management. I hope to bridge that gap with this book. The information presented in *The Woman's Guide to Managing Migraine* should help facilitate improved dialogue between you and your health-care provider and result in improved treatment. Ultimately, the goal is for you to live as headache-free as possible. Let's get started!

Susan Hutchinson, M.D.
Director and Founder,
Orange County Migraine and Headache Center
Irvine, California
April 7, 2012

The Woman's Guide to Managing Migraine

An Introduction to Menstrual Migraine

H EADACHE IS AN ALMOST UNIVERSAL CONDITION. Almost everyone has had a headache at some point. However, there remains a big difference between mild tension headaches compared to more disabling migraine-type headaches.

The focus of this book is on migraine and especially on menstrual migraines. Just how common is migraine in the United States? Let's take a look at prevalence, which refers to the number or percentage of the population that experiences a particular condition in a given year. Physicians and epidemiologists look to prevalence data to understand who is experiencing a condition and whether there are age, gender, or other demographic trends.

A recent study looked at patterns of migraine in a U.S. population of 40,892 men, women, and children who participated in the 2003 National Headache Interview Survey.[1] Migraine prevalence was 17.5% in women and 8.6% in men in the study. The overall prevalence was 13.2%. In both sexes, migraine peaked in the late teens and twenties, and again around 50 years of age. After the age of 10, females were more likely to have migraine than males.[1]

According to these data, which are consistent with several large population-based studies dating back to 1989, 13.2% of the population of the United States is experiencing at least one migraine headache in any given year. This translates to about 30 million adult Americans (age 18 and up) suffering from migraines every year. Of those 30 million migraine sufferers, about 22 million are women.

Migraine tends to follow certain common trends over the lifespan. The 17–18% migraine prevalence for women is an average, and this figure is not constant throughout a woman's life span. Women between the ages of 25 and 55 often experience more migraines than do other women; in particular, migraine prevalence is as high as 25–27% for women aged 30 to 49. Figure 1-1 shows a snapshot of the lifespan of migraine prevalence in women.

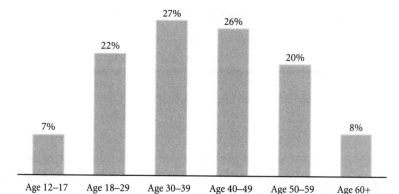

FIGURE 1-1 Migraine Prevalence: US Female Population. Reprinted with permission from Lipton RB, Stewart WF, Diamond S, et al. Prevalence and burden of migraine in the United States: data from the American Migraine Study II. Headache. 2001;41(7):646–657.

The prevalence ratio of females to males is highest during the female reproductive or child-bearing years and is often quoted at 3:1, with many more women having migraines than men. After the age of 42, the prevalence ratio is approximately 2:1 for women compared to men.[1]

❖

Why are prevalence data important? They help to show just how common migraine is. If you are a female between the ages of 25 and 55, there is an approximately 25% chance you have migraine. And if you are reading this book because you tend to get headaches around your period, I estimate a more than 75% chance that your headaches are migraine! You are not alone. Many other women know the pain of migraine and how disabling this condition can be throughout one's life. Here are some of their stories. We will be visiting these women again over the course of this book.

Meet Nancy, a 29-year-old woman. She is an attorney, striving to become a partner in the law practice where she works. Her migraines are becoming more frequent and can last for 2–3 days, especially when she is on her period. Recently, she woke up vomiting, with a very bad headache, and had to miss work for 2 days. Her male colleagues were not very happy that they had to do some of her work in her absence. She is worried that she may have a bad headache on a day when she is scheduled to go to court. In fact, she is getting so worried about getting a headache that she is not enjoying life, even when she does not have a headache. She has begun to date Keith, a 36-year-old attorney, who has made partner at a different law firm. He does not understand why she can't just lie down until her headache goes away.

❖

Lisa is a 25-year-old teacher working in a classroom of 30 high-energy second graders. She loves her work but migraines are causing major problems for her students and her career. If she has a mild to moderate headache, she simply takes Excedrin (acetaminophen-aspirin-caffeine combination) and goes to work. However, around her period, she may wake up with a headache that is so severe she can barely lift her head off her pillow. Her head is pounding, she is nauseated, and the morning light is unbearable. On these days, she has to call in sick. Her doctor has prescribed Imitrex (sumatriptan) tablets for her, but she "saves" them for her bad migraines so she won't run out of the nine Imitrex tablets a month that her insurance allows. She is using up all her sick days and is worried that she may lose her job. When she complains to her husband, Rick, he simply tells her she needs to exercise more and learn to handle stress better. He has never had bad headaches.

❖

Melanie is a 35-year-old mother of two; her children are 7 and 5 years old. She always wanted to be a mother but now wonders if she made a mistake in having kids. Her husband travels a lot, and she often feels like a single parent. When she gets near her period, she suffers from unbearable headaches and does not even want to get out of bed. She finds that she is irritable with her kids and often yells at them during a headache attack. She yells at them to turn the TV volume down and to quit running around their house. She even has them take their shoes off and instructs them to tip-toe around the house when her head is pounding. Depression is now setting in because she feels guilty that she yells at her kids and gets so irritable with them. Her husband, Tom, gets frustrated when he comes home from a trip, and she just wants to go to bed and lie down with an ice pack on her head. He feels as if he does not have the wife he married. Her headaches often start 1–2 days before her period and can last for days; sometimes a headache can last for 1 week straight.

❖

Beth is a 19-year-old single college student struggling to keep up her GPA. She is considering applying to medical school, but lately her headaches make it almost impossible to study during the week of her period. She is dating; she visited her gynecologist's office to be put on birth control pills to help regulate her periods and for birth control. She has been dating Ryan for 3 months, and they are now sexually active. She was hoping the birth control pill would help her period-related headaches but now they are worse. In addition, she suffers from severe premenstrual symptoms (PMS) including mood swings, bloating, and breast tenderness before her period. She called her gynecologist's office, and the nurse told her to stop taking the birth control pills since her headaches have gotten worse.

❖

Theresa is a 40-year-old woman in the middle of a messy divorce. Her husband was having an affair over a 2-year period. She has two teenage sons and is struggling to pay the bills. She works part-time for a real estate firm. She is getting sinus headaches with her period every month; they are making it difficult for her to function. She is trying over-the-counter antihistamines and decongestants, but they do not completely relieve her period-related sinus headaches.

❖

Christy is a divorced 47-year-old woman with irregular periods and hard-to-predict migraine headaches. When she was younger, her migraines were easier to predict since her periods were regular. Now, she feels as if her life and headaches are totally out of control. She works in sales and is on commission; in recent months, she has not met her quota and is worried about her job. She is on several Internet dating sites but has not had very good luck lately with the men she has been meeting. Her 21-year-old daughter, Alexis, lives with her and goes to a local community college. A son, Brian, is 18 and in his senior year of high school. Alexis has been having headaches with her period and may miss classes for 1–2 days a month.

❖

Kate is 55 years old, happily married to Bob, and the mother of three grown children. She had migraines for many years, sometimes with her period. She is now completely menopausal and her headaches occur less often, but she now struggles with hot flashes, night sweats, and insomnia. She is considering estrogen but is afraid it will aggravate her migraines. She is also afraid of increasing her risk of breast cancer. She works as an office manager in a busy dental practice. One of the dental hygienists, Claire, calls in sick 2–3 days a month because of migraines. This is a major disruption to all the patients who are booked with Claire on those days. Claire has used up all her sick time. As office manager, Kate is struggling with how to handle this situation. The two owners of the practice are frustrated with Claire and are asking Kate to do something about this situation.

112 MILLION BEDRIDDEN DAYS

Nancy, Lisa, Melanie, Beth, Theresa, Christy, and Kate represent many of the patients in my practice who I see for menstrual migraine. Each has a unique story to tell, and I hope their stories will help you to find the path that will help you find relief for your menstrual migraines.

Through the prevalence data discussed in this chapter, we can begin to understand the impact of migraine in society. The disability associated with migraine causes great disruption in family and work life. Not only does the individual who has migraine suffer during an attack, countless coworkers and family members also suffer, in different ways. Migraine affects one out of every four households in America. There are stories like Nancy's, Lisa's, Melanie's, Beth's, Theresa's, Christy's, and Kate's playing out every day in this country.

Migraine is often a life-long condition. The World Health Organization ranks migraine 19th among all causes of "years lived with disability." Migraine is a common reason for disability claims and is often the reason that patients request family medical leave. Many sufferers are afraid they will lose their jobs because of absences. According to one study, migraine is responsible for 112 million bedridden days per year in the United States,[2] and, in another—a large population-based study called the American Migraine Study—51.1% of women and 38.1% of men with migraine experienced the equivalent of 6 or more lost workdays per year.[3] It is not uncommon for one of my patients to tell me "I want to cut my head off..."

Prevalence of Menstrual Headaches (Menstrual Migraine)

Between 21 and 22 million women in the United States suffer from migraine every year. Thirteen million of them, about 60%, have a hormonal connection between their headaches and their menstrual cycles, and these women suffer from menstrual migraine. This hormonal connection can happen whenever a woman's estrogen and progesterone levels change. In particular, the drop in estrogen and progesterone that occurs just before menstruation is considered the key trigger for menstrual headache.

The time in a woman's life when migraine is most likely to occur—her 20s through her early 50s—represents her peak career earning-power years and child-rearing years. The associated disability can have disastrous consequences, financial and emotional. Figure 1-2 illustrates the breakdown of migraine prevalence.

In contrast, only 7 to 8 million men in the United States suffer from migraine every year. The simple reason for the disparity between genders is the different behavior between dominant "male" (e.g., testosterone) and "female" (e.g., estrogen, progesterone) hormones. Testosterone levels do not cycle and change as estrogen and progesterone levels do. We will explore the relationship between estrogen and headache more deeply in Chapter 6.

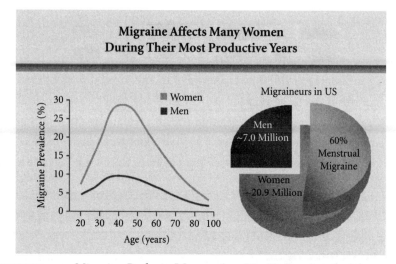

FIGURE 1-2 Migraine Peaks in Women Age 30–49. Reprinted with permission from Lipton RB, Stewart WF, Diamond S, et al Prevalence and burden of migraine in the United States: data from the American Migraine Study II. Headache. 2001;41:646–657 and Mannix LK, Calhoun AH. Menstrual Migraine., Curr Treat Options Neurol. 2004;6(6):489–498.

To better understand the impact of the prevalence of menstrual migraine, it's important to clearly define what menstrual migraine is.

Not "Just a Headache"

A few years ago, Theresa asked her small Bible Study Women's Group to pray for the "sinus" headaches she was getting every month with menstruation. I explained to her that we would pray for her, but I felt confident that what she was experiencing was menstrual migraines. I recommended that she ask her healthcare provider for a migraine-specific medication like a triptan (more about triptans in the Chapter

5). She came back to Bible Study several weeks later with good news: Her doctor had given her a prescription for Imitrex (sumatriptan, a migraine-specific medication), and she finally had an effective treatment plan for her monthly headaches.

> **Box 1-1**
>
> Many women mistakenly think it is normal to suffer "period headaches," thinking that not much can be done. I have heard of male gynecologists who tell their patients, "Honey, it is just a headache. Live with it." In so many of these cases, physicians who give this kind of advice are wrong.

Menstrual migraine is a disabling headache that occurs sometime between 2 days before and 3 days into a woman's period. A physician will consider the pattern menstrual migraine if it occurs in at least two-thirds (66%) of a woman's cycles.[4]

Are all monthly headaches menstrual migraine? In almost every case, the answer is yes. It may be possible for a woman to occasionally suffer from a tension headache with menstruation, but in my experience, I find this to be rare.

Premenstrual Syndrome and Headache: What's the Connection?

Premenstrual syndrome (PMS) refers to all the physical and emotional symptoms that often accompany the time leading up to a women's menstrual period. Symptoms like bloating and breast tenderness are common, but a disabling headache is not. This is not necessarily common knowledge. Many women accept monthly headaches as part of PMS and never have their headaches evaluated as a separate condition.

Box 1-2

Menstrual migraine (monthly disabling headaches with menstruation) is a completely separate condition from premenstrual syndrome (PMS). A woman can have both conditions or suffer from just one. Never accept a disabling monthly headache as simply part of PMS. Monthly headaches deserve evaluation and treatment apart from PMS.

Significantly, the majority of women with menstrual migraine have *menstrual-related migraine*. This refers to women who have migraines during times not related to their menstrual cycles *in addition* to their menstrual migraines. Data suggest that 46% of female migraine patients show this pattern.[5] In contrast, only 14% of women migraine patients suffer from pure menstrual migraine, in which they only have

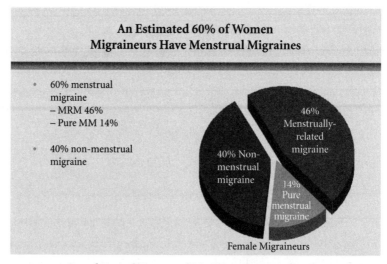

FIGURE 1-3 Prevalence of Menstrual Migraine. Reprinted with permission from Mannix LK, Calhoun AH. Menstrual migraine. Curr Treat Options Neurol. 2004;6(6):489–498 and Lay CL, Mascellino AM. Menstrual migraine:diagnosis and treatment. Curr Pain Headache Rep. 2001;5(2):195–199.

migraines during their menstrual time of the month.[5] The remaining 40% of women with migraine have no clear association between their migraine headaches and their menstrual cycles (see Figure 1-3).

As a headache specialist, understanding this prevalence data helps me to diagnose patients who come to my practice and to make the best treatment decisions for each particular patient. Prevalence data can also assist patients in determining what type of headache pattern they might have and what treatment approaches may help. To illustrate, let's learn more about Beth's story.

Beth's disabling headache typically begins 1–2 days before her period and lasts for 3–5 days. She estimates this headache happens with 90% of her menstrual cycles. She occasionally reports a headache not related to menstruation that is very mild compared to her "period-related headaches." She also gets moody and tearful before her period; her gynecologist prescribed Zoloft (sertraline) for her to take for a diagnosis of premenstrual dysphoric disorder (PMDD). She was told that her headaches may improve with Zoloft. After several months, she reports back to her doctor's office. She is still suffering from disabling period-related headaches despite taking Excedrin Migraine (acetaminophen-aspirin-caffeine).

Prevalence data would strongly suggest menstrual migraine as Beth's diagnosis. Her headache should not be considered as simply part of her premenstrual symptoms. Her premenstrual dysphoric disorder (PMDD) and PMS symptoms would be expected to improve with Zoloft (sertraline), but not her migraines. She needs migraine-specific medication for her disabling headaches, such as a triptan (see Chapter 5 for an in-depth discussion of treatment). Keeping a headache calendar will help determine if Beth suffers from menstrual-related migraines, which we know from prevalence data to be more common, or from pure menstrual migraine.

On follow-up, Beth's headache calendar showed only an occasional, mild, tension-type headache during the weeks she was not on her period, and she was able to take Tylenol (acetaminophen) or Excedrin for those headaches. They were not associated with any nausea or sensitivity to light. She was diagnosed with pure menstrual migraine.

Now let's look at Melanie, the mother of two, who suffers from severe menstrual migraines that can last for 5–7 days. Her physician encourages her to keep a headache diary for 3 months. It shows one to two headaches a week, including the bad headache the week of her period. Some of her nonmenstrual headaches can be severe; triggers include lack of sleep and stress. She has menstrual migraine but, unlike Beth, Melanie has menstrual-related migraine as well. Management for Beth can focus on her one bad week of the month. Management for Melanie will need to focus on all her migraines, including those that occur apart from her period.

What Happens as Women Get Older?

Good news: The prevalence of migraine goes down after age 50. In particular, for women who go through menopause spontaneously (their ovaries are not surgically removed), two-thirds will find their migraines go away or improve dramatically. As we've seen, and as we discuss in more detail in later chapters, hormones and migraine in many women are intimately connected.

For men, also, the prevalence of migraine decreases with advancing age.

Other Types of Headache

Women often come into my practice thinking they have *cluster headache*. This is often because they see a pattern where their headaches "cluster together" in a concentrated period of 5–7 days (for example, with menstruation), followed by a headache-free period of 3 weeks.

On further questioning and evaluation, they usually end up with a diagnosis of migraine. The prevalence of cluster headache is very low compared to that of migraine—only 0.1–0.4% of the population, compared to 13% for migraine. It is the only primary headache that is more common in men than in women; in fact, the ratio is 7:1, in favor of males. It is characterized by a boring, piercing pain behind one eye, tearing in the eye that hurts, and drooping of the eyelid on the affected side. It is often referred to as the "suicide headache," based on its extreme pain. In contrast to a migraine attack, during which the sufferer wants to be in a dark, quiet room, the cluster headache patient is usually pacing, agitated, and often hitting his or her head into a wall.

As the name "cluster" implies, someone with this kind of headache can go for weeks, months, and even years without a headache, but during a "cluster" episode, the headache can occur several times a day and can last for weeks or months. It then will go away for long stretches at a time.

In contrast, menstrual migraine is usually much more predictable. It occurs with almost every menstrual cycle and does not go away for months or years.

BOX 1-3

Prevalence data suggest that most women with disabling headaches have migraines. Cluster headache is very rare in women.

Where Does Tension Headache Fit in with Migraine?

Tension headache is an almost universal condition that almost everyone has experienced at some time. Tension headache, by definition, is only mild to moderate in severity, is not associated with nausea, and only occasionally causes sensitivity to light or noise. Most individuals with tension headache "power through" them and take either nothing or something over-the-counter like Excedrin, aspirin, Aleve (naproxen) or Motrin (ibuprofen). Migraine sufferers may well have tension headaches in addition to their migraines. Common triggers for tension headache include stress, lack of exercise, and neck-related issues from sitting in front of a computer for long stretches of time. There is no reliable prevalence data on tension headache since it is believed to be an almost universal condition.

You Are Not Alone

Over half of women with migraine suffer from menstrual migraine. For many, the menstrual migraines are the most disabling of all their migraine attacks. A trial involving more than 1,000 women showed that those with menstrual migraine had significant disability involving social activity (84%), household chores (81%), and work (45%).[6]

Menstrual migraine, by definition, will go away when a woman stops having periods. The average age of menopause is 50–52. This is good news for patients like Beth, Melanie, Nancy, Lisa, Kate, Christy, and Theresa, although most of them have many years until they reach menopause.

The rest of this book is dedicated to helping women, like those we met in this chapter, to shed the burden of menstrual migraine in their lives. Your story may be similar to that of one of these women. We all have unique stories to tell.

References

1. Victor TW, Hu X, Campbell JC, et al. Migraine prevalence by age and sex in the United States: as life-span study. Cephalalgia 2010; 30(9): 1065–1072. Epub Mar 12 2010.
2. Hu XH, Markson LE, Lipton RB, et al. Burden of migraine in the United States: disability and economic costs. Arch Intern Med. 1999; 159: 813–818.

3. Stewart WF, Lipton RB, Simon D. Work-related disability: results from the American Migraine Study. Cephalalgia. 1996; 16: 231–238.

4. International Headache Society. The international classification of headache disorders. Cephalalgia. 2004; 24(suppl 1): 1–151.

5. Mannix LK, Calhoun AH. Menstrual migraine. Curr Treat Options Neurol. 2004; 6(6): 489–498.

6. Couturier EG, Bomhof MA, Neven AK, et al. Menstrual migraine in a representative Dutch population sample: prevalence, disability, and treatment. Cephalalgia. 2003; 23(4): 302–308.

2

What Causes Headache in Women?

BETH COMES IN FOR A VISIT TO THE STUDENT HEALTH Center on her college campus. She is frustrated with the disabling headaches she gets with her period every month. She tries so hard to exercise, eat healthy, get enough sleep, and yet it is not enough. The doctor diagnoses menstrual migraine. Beth begins to cry; she asks the doctor, "What am I doing wrong? Why am I getting these headaches?"

The cause of headache in women cannot be answered with a simple explanation. Many factors are involved; in addition, research continues to expand our knowledge of the cause of headache. As in other chapters, here we will focus on the cause of migraine, including menstrual migraine, in women. If you are not sure if you have migraine, you may want to skip ahead to Chapter 3, take the "headache quiz," then come back to this chapter to learn more.

Research indicates that most migraine patients have inherited a genetic predisposition to the disorder. Most individuals who have migraines (also known as *migraineurs*) will have one or more family members who have migraines as well. It is often useful to know your family history for any and all headache issues and other family members' experiences. Some may report getting frequent "sinus" or tension headaches, but such headaches may actually be migraines. For example, my mother often says we tend to get "sinus headaches" in our family. But what my mother has called "sinus" headaches are actually migraines.

A team of international researchers has recently identified the first-ever genetic link to common migraine (*common migraine* refers to migraine without *aura,* and it is the most common type of migraine that occurs). This team of researchers looked at genetic data from 50,000 people from Finland, Germany, and the Netherlands. They found that individuals with a particular DNA variant on chromosome 8 have a significantly greater risk for developing migraine.[1] Specifically, the variant on chromosome 8 occurs between two genes, *PGCP* and *MTDH/AEG-1.* This variant regulates levels of glutamate, which is a chemical in the brain that helps nerve cells communicate. The results of the study suggest that a buildup of this glutamate may be associated with an increased susceptibility to common migraine. Researchers have described genetic mutations related to rare and more extreme forms of migraine, such as *hemiplegic migraine* (described in detail in the Chapter 3), but this is the first time a team has identified a genetic link for common migraine. This breakthrough research may lead to new and better migraine prevention. For example, a migraine preventive could be designed to lower levels of glutamate.

❖

Beth, sitting in the Student Health Center of her university, is wondering what she is doing wrong to get these disabling menstrual headaches. Her physician tells her the truth: She has done nothing wrong. It is more likely that she inherited the susceptibility to migraine from her mother or her father's side of the family, or from both. Although there are many parts of our life we can control, like our health habits, we cannot control our genetic makeup, which was determined at the time of conception.

When asked about family history, Beth admits that her mother got bad headaches with her period when she was Beth's age. Her younger sister seems to be fine and is not troubled with headaches. Beth is reassured that she did nothing wrong to cause her headaches, but expresses her frustration and worry that these headaches will make it difficult for her to make the grades she needs to get into medical school.

The "Ferrari" Brain

What is it that migraine individuals inherit? What is the result of this genetic variant that may be linked to common migraine?

As a migraine sufferer, my favorite metaphor is of the "Ferrari" brain. I like to explain that the individual who has migraine has inherited a brain that tends to be very sensitive to internal or external changes. Such changes can set off a cascade of events (discussed in Chapter 3) that cause the migraine episode. The brain of someone with migraine is like a Ferrari sports car: a very fine-tuned system. The brain of an individual without migraine is like a Ford or Chevrole and requires less maintenance. In general, an expensive sports car requires more attention to keep it in its high performance state than does a less expensive car. As migraine sufferers, we need to carefully maintain our bodies and brains to minimize the disruptions and changes that can cause a migraine. (We will talk about proper "maintenance" in more detail in the chapters devoted to treatment.)

The sensitivity of the migraine brain can be difficult for others to understand. Lisa, the 25-year-old teacher, and Melanie, the 35-year-old mother of two, both feel that their husbands do not understand the sensitivity they have to their surroundings. For example, Lisa does not enjoy going to the beach for the day since the sun and heat can trigger a migraine attack. Melanie does not want to schedule a family vacation around her period as she may end up staying in the hotel room the whole time. Both husbands are frustrated because they have to change their plans based on their wives' headaches. Melanie's husband, Tom, gets stuck watching the kids when Melanie has what he thinks of as her "period headaches," and he has to cancel tee time with his buddies. He just wants her to get better, and he does not understand why she can't find a treatment plan that will work. He has begun searching the Internet for solutions. Lisa's husband, Rick, ends up going to the beach by himself to surf and play beach volleyball. Lisa stays home and works on crafts and indoor projects but is annoyed that her headaches cause her to miss out on going to the beach with her husband.

The Origins of a Migraine

For a migraine to develop, a change has to occur, either inside the body or in the environment around the body. Often, several factors come together to cause that particular migraine. Most women who have migraine find that they are extra vulnerable to their migraine triggers during certain times of their cycle. This is one of the reasons that it is important for all women with recurring headaches to keep a calendar or diary of their headaches, taking into account when their period occurs. The first and last day of menstruation should always be recorded on a headache calendar or diary. Beth is instructed to begin keeping a diary of all her headaches, not just those that are menstrual-related, and to watch for patterns in what occurs in the 24 hours leading up to any of her headaches. She knows her hormones are a cause, but she needs to track other triggers or causes to better understand and help her headaches. The leading causes of migraine in women migraine patients include:

- Changes in hormone levels, especially estrogen
- Stress
- Changes in barometric pressure (weather changes)
- High altitude
- Sun exposure, heat
- Food triggers (e.g., preservatives such as monosodium glutamate [MSG] or sulfites)

- Alcohol
- Excessive caffeine
- Skipping meals
- Changes in blood sugar (e.g., hypoglycemia)
- Not enough protein
- Lack of sleep or disrupted sleep
- Neck muscle tightness
- Some medications, such as synthetic estrogen

The most frequent cause of migraine in women is hormonal. Specifically, the times in a woman's cycle that make her most vulnerable to getting a migraine attack are those times when estrogen levels are changing. Figure 2-1 shows what happens to estrogen and progesterone during a woman's menstrual cycle. Notice the drop in estrogen at the end of the cycle as a woman gets close to menstruation.

Times of hormonal change include:

- During and around the time of the period, when estrogen levels are low
- At ovulation (a rise or peak in estrogen followed by a drop)

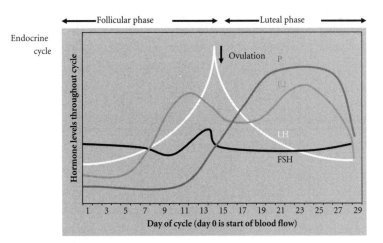

FIGURE 2-1 Hormone Levels During the Menstrual Cycle. Reprinted with permission from Silberstein SD, Lipton RB, Goadsby PJ. *Headache in Clinical Practice*, 2nd ed. New York: Martin Dunitz; 2002: 102.

- Postpartum (after delivery), when estrogen levels drop dramatically
- Perimenopause (when estrogen levels are wildly fluctuating); this is typically in a woman's 40s and early 50s)
- During the placebo week of contraceptive products like the birth control pill, the vaginal contraceptive ring (NuvaRing [etonogestrel/ethinyl estradiol), or the birth control patch (Ortho Evra [norelgestromin, ethinyl estradiol])
- When hormonal replacement medication begins to wear off, such as at the end of an estrogen patch's lifespan (when blood levels of estrogen are getting lower)
- Surgical menopause (removal of ovaries)

The graph in Figure 2-2 illustrates the high frequency of migraine during times when estrogen levels drop in a woman's cycle.

In Figure 2-2, notice the increase in migraine during the days of low estrogen blood levels. Higher levels of estrogen during a woman's cycle appear to protect against migraine occurrence; lower levels increase the chance of a migraine attack in susceptible women.

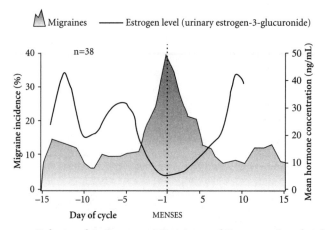

FIGURE 2-2 Relationship Between Migraine and Estrogen Level. Adapted with permission from Silberstein SD, Elkind AH, Schreiber C, Keywood C. A randomized trial of frovatriptan for the intermittent prevention of menstrual migraine. *Neurology*. 2004; 63:261–269.

Knowing this connection between our hormone levels and migraine occurrence can help with treatment. Trying to maintain an even estrogen level can be very helpful in reducing the burden of migraine in the more than 60% of women migraine patients who have this hormonal trigger. This treatment approach will be discussed in great detail in Chapter 6.

Changes in progesterone levels also occur during a woman's menstrual cycle. However, studies do not indicate a clear relationship between changes in progesterone levels and migraine occurrence. This will also be discussed in more detail in Chapter 6.

Nonhormonal causes of migraine are many, including stress, lack of sleep, preservatives (such as MSG and sulfites), and changes in barometric pressure. These all represent an internal or external change in a susceptible individual's normal routine. Any change, even a small one, can trigger the cascade of events that characterize migraine. The identification and management of nonhormonal migraine triggers will be discussed in more detail in Chapter 7.

Beth still has questions about her migraines. She understands that she inherited a genetic predisposition to migraine from her mother. She is beginning to be aware of her own risk factors or triggers, such as her period, stress, and lack of sleep. However, she still wants to understand what is happening in her body to cause the headache and, in her case, the associated nausea and sensitivity to light. She did some reading and came across the term "vascular headache" to describe migraine. She knows *vascular* means blood vessels, and she asks, "Is this the reason I feel pounding in my head during a migraine? Is it the blood vessels getting bigger?"

What is causing Beth's pounding headache? What actually occurs inside our body during a migraine attack?
If you look through old medical textbooks, you'll notice, as Beth did, that migraine headache was often referred to as "vascular headache." The common thinking used to be that there was an initial period in a migraine when the blood vessels in the brain would constrict or get

smaller, responding to a decrease in blood flow; this was followed by a period when the blood vessels would dilate and grow larger, with an increase in blood flow. The initial constriction of the blood vessels was thought to account for the aura that some patients get before their headache. (Aura will be discussed in more detail in Chapter 3.) In the past, it was believed that the reason many migraine attacks are associated with a throbbing or pulsating feeling in the temple and head area was owing to blood vessels are getting larger with more blood flow. However, new research has shown that migraine headaches are more than "vascular"; they are "neurovascular." As we will see, the key to understanding what causes a migraine is to understand that the nervous system is very much involved in a migraine attack.

The migraine headache emerges at the end of a sequence of events occurring in both the blood vessels and nervous system of our body. Researchers and specialists think that the sequence of events plays out like this:

1. An internal or external change disrupts a normally function-ing nervous system in an individual who has a history of migraines. A common change is the drop in estrogen that occurs just before a menstrual period. In women who are sus-ceptible to migraines, this drop in estrogen causes an inflam-matory response.

The next steps in the sequence involve our cranial nerves. There are 12 cranial nerves in our nervous system; they function to sup-ply sensory and motor sensations for the head and neck. When an inflammatory response is launched, the fifth cranial nerve, also known as the *trigeminal nerve*, is responsible for the activa-tion of the peripheral nervous system. This activation takes place in the scalp, head, and facial area. The fifth cranial or trigeminal nerve has branches on both the right and left sides of our faces (Figure 2-3).

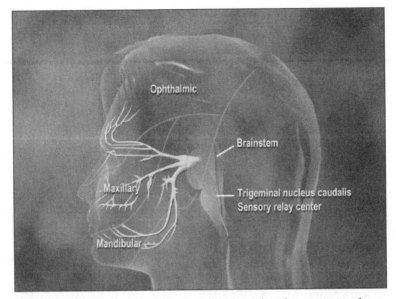

FIGURE 2-3 Trigeminal Nerve Location. Adapted with permission from Primary Care Network.

2. The trigeminal nerve can become activated or inflamed on one side or both sides of the face. As it becomes activated, it can cause facial pain and pressure, including pain behind the eyes. Facial pain over the cheeks and even the jaws may occur. These pain locations can be explained by the distribution of the trigeminal nerve, as shown in Figure 2-3.

3. The trigeminal nerve activation then causes the release of chemicals, often called *neurotransmitters*, which can cause blood vessels in the area to become inflamed, enlarge, and begin to throb or pound. These neurotransmitters include substance P, calcitonin gene-related peptide, and prostaglandins.

4. The inflammation spreads from the peripheral nerves to the brainstem and continues to travel up to the brain itself. It is as if the migraine has a life of its own, continuing to progress and worsen if a treatment does not break the sequence of events.

5. As the migraine progresses and moves centrally to the brainstem and brain itself, it becomes harder and harder to treat.

In fact, there is often a point in a migraine attack at which no oral medication can stop it. The individual may need to resort to an injection, a nasal spray, or an intravenous form of treatment. This will be discussed in more detail in Chapter 5.

The release of the chemicals that cause inflammation (step 3) accounts for the pounding and throbbing that is characteristic of migraine headache attacks. This also explains the worsening of pain with exertion, such as occurs with bending over, going up stairs, coughing, or rapid head movement. This worsening with exertion is not present in tension-type headache and helps to diagnose the type of headache that is present.

The part of the brainstem that becomes activated during a migraine is very near the area of the brainstem that control sinus congestion, nasal congestion, and tear glands in the eye. If this area becomes activated, it can lead to the congestion and tearing that many individuals experience during a migraine attack. Also nearby in this region are the nerves that go to the back of the head and neck. This helps explain the pain in the neck and back of the head that many experience during attacks. Figure 2-4 illustrates some of the activity that occurs in the brainstem during a migraine attack.

The center for nausea and vomiting also is near the part of the brainstem that becomes activated during a migraine. The theory is that because this center often becomes activated during a migraine attack, it then leads to the nausea and vomiting commonly experienced with a migraine.

The explanation I have given, showing the sequence of events that cause pain and other associated symptoms during a migraine, is an introduction to the science behind the migraine. Sources that give more detail on what causes a migraine and what is occurring during a migraine attack can be found in neurology medical textbooks and articles published in headache journals. In addition, more information is available by accessing some of the resources in the appendix.

One Nerve Pathway, Multiple Symptoms, Multiple Manifestations of Migraine

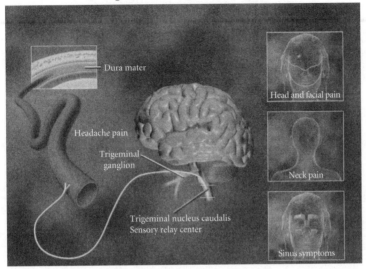

FIGURE 2-4 Migraine Activity. Adapted with permission from Primary Care Network.

What Causes Aura?

Kate, the 55-year-old migraine patient we met in Chapter 1, occasionally gets aura before her migraines. Her aura symptoms include a shimmering in her visual field that she describes as heat waves and flashes of light. She may also experience tingling around her mouth. Usually, these aura symptoms last for 20–30 minutes, then her headache occurs. She wants to know what is causing her aura.

Aura is experienced in only 10–14% of migraine patients. It is thought to be due to an event called *cortical spreading depression*, in which a wave of electrical activity moves across the cerebral cortex, the main part of the brain.[2] This wave of electrical activity causes changes in blood flow and often affects the part of the brain involved in vision, the occipital lobe. Other parts of the brain can be affected as well and cause other aura symptoms. For example, Kate's mother experienced tingling and numbness in her hand, moving up her arm, and then up into her face during her aura. This symptom can be explained by cortical spreading depression affecting the parietal lobes of her brain, in particular, those parts involved with somatosensory processing. In some cases, cortical spreading depression can affect the motor section of the frontal lobe involved with voluntary movement; in this case, the individual may experience weakness of the arms or legs and difficulty with coordination. However, the majority of women and men with migraine do not have aura. The stages of a migraine are explained in detail in Chapter 3.

BOX 2-1

Migraine is caused by a disruption in our neurovascular system and involves changes in both blood vessels and elements of our nervous system. The change can come from the body itself, such as a change in estrogen levels in women, or it can come from the external environment, such as a change in barometric pressure or exposure to a bright light. The key to understanding the migraine pathway is to be aware of the involvement of the trigeminal nerve, nearby blood vessels, and pathways leading to the brainstem and the brain itself.

Recent published research indicates that there may be a genetic link associated with migraine. This link may involve a DNA variant on chromosome 8, and it may help explain why some individuals suffer from migraine and others do not. Learning more about this genetic link may lead to a greater understanding of what causes migraine and may lead to more effective treatment.

References

1. ScienceDaily. August 30, 2010. Accessed September 9, 2010. http://www.sciencedaily.com/releases/2010/08/100829201954. htm

2. Lauritzen M. Pathophysiology of the migraine aura. The spreading depression theory. Brain 1994; 117 199–210.

3

What Kind of Headache Do I Have?

A LMOST EVERYONE HAS HAD A HEADACHE AT SOME time in his or her life. Tension headache is the most common form of headache; however, by definition, tension headache only leads to mild to moderate disability. It is not the headache that drives you to go to your doctor's office or the emergency room. In contrast, migraine headache is often associated with moderate to severe disability and is a leading cause of missed days from work and interference with social activities and daily living. If you are reading this book, your headaches are most likely interfering with the quality of your life.

Headache can be divided into *primary* and *secondary* forms. Primary headaches are those in which the headache is the problem and there is no secondary cause, such as a brain tumor. Secondary headaches are headaches in which there is an underlying reason for the headache, such as a brain tumor or meningitis. Here, we'll focus mostly on the different types of primary headache.

Tension

A tension headache is best described as a tightening or pressing feeling around the head, like a tight band. Often, the pain is concentrated in the forehead area. There is no nausea. In general, those with tension headache continue to work, go to school, and carry on activities of daily life. One of the distinguishing characteristics of tension headache compared to migraine is that there is no worsening of head pain with movement or activity. In several published studies, 72–84% of episodic tension-type headache sufferers reported no worsening of their headaches with activity.[1,2] Many tension headache sufferers may take an over-the-counter analgesic like Tylenol (acetaminophen), aspirin, or a combination analgesic such as Excedrin (aspirin-acetaminophen-caffeine), or they take nothing at all. This type of headache does not drive individuals to seek help at doctor's offices or in the emergency room.

Cluster

The cluster headache is often referred to as the "suicide headache" because it can be so severe that sufferers feel like committing suicide. Indeed, there have been reports of violent self-harm because of the severe intensity of the pain.[3] The attack can begin as a vague discomfort but rapidly increases to maximal intensity in 9 minutes in 86% of patients.[4] Characteristics of this headache can include pacing about the room, banging one's head into the wall, and being extremely agitated. The cluster headache patient usually complains of a boring, piercing pain behind one eye, tearing of the same eye, and often drooping of the eyelid on the affected side. The cluster headache usually lasts 30 minutes to 2 hours and occurs in a range of one attack every other day to eight attacks daily. Attacks tend to occur at the same time during the day or night. Most patients report a predictable attack that wakes them from sleep, often 90 minutes after going to sleep.[5] As the name implies, cluster headache tends to "cluster" together for weeks or months in the affected individual, and then may go away for months or years. This headache affects a very small percentage of the population—only 0.05–0.4%—and it is seven times more likely to affect men than women. Chances are, if you are a woman reading this book, you don't have cluster headache. Keep in mind that you may have headaches that "cluster" together, but they are usually migraine headaches.

Migraine

A migraine is an episodic, disabling headache often described as a throbbing, pulsating, "sick" headache that is more common in women than men. Nausea, vomiting, sensitivity to light and noise, and worsening with activity are all associated with migraine. Predictable triggers, such as a woman's period (menses), help support the diagnosis of migraine. Approximately 30 million Americans suffer from migraine in any given year in this country; about 22.5 million are women. This represents 13% of the adult population as a whole, 18% women and 6% men.

You may have already identified which headache you have. If not, you may find the flowchart in Table 3-1 helpful.

It is always a good idea to have your headache diagnosis confirmed by your physician or healthcare provider. To make the correct headache diagnosis, your doctor will use established guidelines formed by the International Classification of Headache Disorders. These headache diagnosis guidelines are well-known to those in the headache field but are often not familiar to many primary care providers who see a myriad of health care issues every day. Awareness of the criteria and the knowledge of how they apply to your headaches can help you be a better advocate for yourself.

TABLE 3-1 What Type of Headache Do You Have?

Do your headaches interfere with your ability to function?

Yes—Migraine or Cluster
No—Tension

Do your headaches

Peak in 9 minutes?
Last 15 minutes to 3 hours if unsuccessfully treated?
Are they always one-sided, with tearing of eye or drooping of the eyelid on the same side as the pain?
Are you restless and agitated during an attack?
Yes—Cluster
No—Migraine

Do your headaches

Last 30 minutes to 72 hours if untreated or not treated successfully?
Is there any nausea with headache attacks and/or sensitivity to light with headache attacks?
Is the pain moderate to severe if untreated successfully?
Is there worsening of head pain with movement?
Yes—Migraine
No—Cluster

Do your headaches

Occur with your menstruation in at least 2 out of 3 cycles?
Occur in the -2 to +3 time of your cycle (2 days before menses up to third day of menses, with Day 1 equal to the first day of flow)?
Yes—Menstrual migraine
If yes, do your headaches
Only occur with menstruation?
Yes—Pure menstrual migraine
No—Menstrual-related migraine

International Headache Society. The International Classification of Headache Disorders, 2nd ed. *Cephalalgia.* 2004;24(Suppl 1):9–160.

BOX 3-1   Many Tension or Sinus Headaches Are Actually Migraine Headaches

Why have I devoted so much space in this book to helping you get the correct diagnosis? Unfortunately, we know from several large population-based studies that approximately half of all migraine patients in the United States have been misdiagnosed with sinus or tension headache. If approximately 30 million Americans suffer from migraine in this country in any given year, then about 15 million may not even know they have migraine. My hope is that readers of this book will be empowered to pursue getting the right diagnosis—so that you can get the best possible treatment and care.

The ID Migraine Screening Tool

The simplest way to identify if you have migraine is to use one of the many screening tools available. One of my favorites is called the ID Migraine screening tool.[6] Here are the screening questions:
During the last 3 months, have you had any of the following with your headaches?

- Did you feel nauseated or sick to your stomach?
- Did light bother you a lot more than when you don't have headaches?
- Did your headaches limit your ability to work, study, or do what you needed to do for at least 1 day?

If you answered "yes" to two or three of these questions, then you have a strong likelihood of having migraines.

Can an individual have more than one type of headache?

Yes. An individual can have both migraines and tension headaches. Or a person could have both migraines and cluster headache. Conceivably, someone could suffer from all three primary headache types: tension, migraine, and cluster.

International Headache Classification Criteria

For the International Headache Classification criteria for tension-type headache, cluster headache, and migraine with and without aura, please see the Appendix.[7]

Aura

The aura phase of a migraine refers to reversible neurological signs and symptoms; luckily, it should last less than 60 minutes. Most often the aura is visual, but it can include sensory symptoms such as tingling and numbness sensations in the body, especially the extremities, and around the mouth and facial area. Sometimes speech will be slurred. If motor weakness is present, or if the arm or leg cannot be raised, then the migraine is more complicated. For example, there is a type of migraine called *hemiplegic migraine* that involves motor weakness, typically of the arm or leg. This is a much more serious migraine.

A caution: Many migraine sufferers and even some healthcare providers overdiagnose aura. Aura is not the blurry vision or sensitivity to light that is typically part of a migraine attack. These visual symptoms are consistent with a migraine without aura (common migraine) diagnosis. A visual aura is not a fleeting flash of light or a speck of light that only lasts for seconds. To meet the strict definition of aura, the visual symptoms must last for at least 5 minutes. It is important to not overdiagnose aura because aura carries with it a higher risk of stroke and that has implications for estrogen use.

Chronic Daily Headache

A primary headache disorder such as tension or migraine can become frequent enough to fit into a category called *chronic daily headache*. By definition, this is a headache that occurs 15 or more days a month. In migraine sufferers, the distinction between migraine and tension headache is often blurred since the almost daily headache loses the "full flavor" of migraine. The following history is common in chronic daily headache patients like Nancy, the 29-year-old attorney: "I used to get migraines two to three times a month, including with my period. Now I am getting a headache almost every day. My almost-daily headache is not severe as long as I take Excedrin. I still get migraines two to three times a month, including with menstruation, and I need my stronger medication for those."

Nancy's history suggests a diagnosis of chronic migraine, also referred to as *transformed migraine*. This is the most common type of chronic daily headache. An individual like Nancy starts off with an episodic migraine pattern of headache that then it evolves or transforms into a more frequent pattern of occurring 15 or more days a month. Sometimes the change or transformation is caused by or associated with medication overuse (for example, Nancy's increasing use of Excedrin [acetaminophen-aspirin-caffeine]). In other individuals, the headache pattern becomes more frequent without any medication overuse. Life stress and hormonal changes can sometimes cause this pattern change.

Chronic daily headache is often associated with medication overuse. The level of use that is considered medication *overuse* depends on the drug but, in general, medication taken for headache attacks 10 days a month or more than two to three times a week can cause chronic daily headache. This problem of medication overuse does not include medications that are taken daily for migraine prevention or for other conditions such as high blood pressure. Nancy is probably overusing Excedrin as she admits to taking it almost every day. If you have a headache more than 15 days a month, ask yourself:

- What do I take for my almost daily headache?
- Am I taking this medication more than two or three times a week?
- Do I have a headache if I don't take this medication?
- Does this medication relieve the headache at least for a while?

If you are suffering from chronic daily headache and medication overuse, I encourage you to seek out a headache specialist in your area. For help finding one, refer to Chapter 11.

I hope by now you have determined what type of headache you have. If in doubt, use your most severe headaches to make the diagnosis. For example, I may have a patient who has different types of headache; some of her headaches are mild and meet the definition only for tension headache; others are more severe, often associated with nausea and may require her to miss work—these meet the criteria for migraine. Looking at my patient's most severe headaches, I will diagnosis her as a migraine sufferer.

Theresa, the 40-year-old headache sufferer we met in Chapter 1, thought she had sinus headaches, but the diagnosis was menstrual migraine. Sinus headache is not considered a primary headache but a secondary headache because it occurs in response to an underlying cause, in most cases a sinus infection. By definition, once the sinus infection is treated with an appropriate course of antibiotics, the headache should resolve. The only primary headache disorders are those we have discussed in this chapter: tension, cluster, and migraine headaches.

Theresa is not alone. Many headache patients think they are having sinus headaches when they are actually having migraines. Theresa, like many migraine patients, experiences sinus pain and pressure with her headaches. She may have nasal congestion and watery eyes. Just leaning her head forward increases headache pain over the sinus area in her forehead. Studies indicate that 45% of migraine sufferers have at least one autonomic symptom of either nasal congestion or watery eyes with their migraine attacks.[8] Autonomic symptoms are part of our nervous system and primarily are made up of involuntary functions that we do not control such as congestion, watery eyes, heart rate, and breathing. In a large multicenter study of almost 3,000 subjects who were self- or physician-diagnosed with sinus headache, 88% of patients actually had migraine and not sinus headaches.[9]

Another common mistake is diagnosing tension headache instead of migraine. The presence of neck pain often suggests tension headache, but in a published study, neck pain was experienced in 75% of migraine attacks. The neck pain can occur before, during, or after the attack.[10] Patients will often report that their neck pain starts in the back of their head and then moves up to the front and settles in around and behind their eyes. As the headache becomes more disabling and associated with nausea, it builds in intensity; that is when we can diagnosis it as migraine.

BOX 3-2   Is It Migraine?

- Do you have a disabling headache that interferes with your ability to function?
- Is there ever nausea or vomiting with your headache?
- Is there ever sensitivity to light or noise with your headache?
- Are there predictable triggers such as menstruation?

If you answered "yes" to two or more of the above, then chances are you have migraine headaches and not sinus or tension headaches.

Secondary Headache

A headache that occurs because of an underlying cause, such as a brain tumor or an acute sinus infection, is a secondary headache. For these headaches, the underlying cause needs to be identified and treated in order for the headache to go away. Here are some clues that your headache may be a secondary headache:

- Is it the worst headache you have ever had?
- Is this a new-onset headache and are you over the age of 40?
- Is there an underlying condition, such as cancer or HIV?
- Are there also systemic symptoms, such as fever or weight loss?
- Is the onset of headache sudden?
- Is the progressive pattern of headache worsening?
- Are there neurological signs or symptoms, such as visual disturbances lasting longer than 60 minutes, problems with

walking, difficulty with speech, weakness in the arms or legs, or persistent numbness or tingling in the arms or legs?

If you suffer from any of these symptoms, or if you are unsure of your headache diagnosis, I encourage you to see your healthcare provider. In general, a stable pattern of headache for over 6 months with predictable triggers (such as menstruation) points to a primary headache disorder such as migraine. But anyone, including those with migraine, tension, and cluster headache, can get a secondary headache related to aneurysm or brain tumor. Therefore, it is important to stay vigilant and watch the pattern of your headaches. As we'll discuss later, in Chapter 7, the best way to do this is with a headache diary or calendar.

Box 3-3   When Is a Brain Scan Necessary?

On occasion a brain scan such as a computed tomography (CT) or magnetic resonance imaging (MRI) of the brain may be necessary to rule out a secondary headache. Other work-up may include a spinal tap and blood work. Brain scans, blood work, and spinal taps are all done to rule out secondary headaches.

The best way to diagnose a primary headache disorder such as migraine, tension, or cluster headache is by carefully examining the history of the headache attacks. I hope this chapter has helped you feel comfortable with the type of headache or headaches you suffer from—and perhaps reassured. Proper diagnosis is the first step to appropriate and effective treatment, and, from there, a balanced routine that minimizes the impact of migraine on your life.

References

1. Rasmussen BK, Jensen R, Schroll M, et al. Interrelations between migraine and tension-type headache in the general population. Arch Neuro. 1992; 49: 914–918.

2. Jensen R, Rasmussen BK, Pedersen B, et al. Muscle tenderness and pressure pain thresholds in headache. A population study. Pain. 1993; 52: 193–199.
3. Blau JN. Behaviour during a cluster headache. Lancet. 1993; 342: 723–725.
4. Torelli P, Manzoni GC. Pain and behavior in cluster headache. A prospective study and review of the literature. Funct Neuro. 2003; 18: 205–210.
5. Bahra A, May A, Goads PJ. Cluster headache: a prospective clinical study with diagnostic implications. Neurology. 2002; 58: 354–361.
6. Lipton RB, Dodick D, Sadovsky R, et al. A self-administered screener for migraine in primary care: the ID Migraine validation study. Neurology. 2003; 61: 375–382.
7. Headache Classification Committee of the International Headache Society. The international classification of headache disorders, 2nd edition. Cephalalgia. 2004; 24(suppl. 1): 1–160.
8. Barbanti P, Fabbrini G, Pesare M, et al. Unilateral cranial autonomic symptoms in migraine. Cephalalgia. 2002; 22: 256–259.
9. Schreiber CP, Hutchinson S, Webster CJ, et al. Prevalence of migraine in patients with a history of self-reported or physician-diagnosed "sinus" headache. Arch Intern Med. 2004; 164: 1769–1772.
10. Kaniecki RG, Totten TD. Cervalgia in migraine: prevalence, clinical characteristics, and response to treatment. Cephalalgia. 2001; 21: 296–297.

4

Common Associated Conditions

MIGRAINE SUFFERERS OFTEN HAVE TO MANAGE other medical conditions in addition to their migraine attacks. Nineteen-year-old Beth, for example, has premenstrual dysphoric disorder (PMDD) in addition to her menstrual migraines. Many medical conditions are seen more often in a female migraine population than would be seen in the general female population. This association is called *comorbidity*. A comorbid condition refers to two disorders coexisting in one individual and that are more commonly seen than would be expected in the general population.

Common associated conditions (or comorbidities) of migraine include:

- Anxiety
- Childhood abuse
- Depression
- Endometriosis
- Fibromyalgia
- Irritable bowel syndrome
- Obesity
- Premenstrual syndrome, premenstrual dysphoric disorder

- Posttraumatic stress disorder (PTSD)
- Sleep disorders
- Stroke

Knowing which medical conditions are commonly associated with migraine will help you select the right treatment plan, including medication. As you read this chapter, I encourage you to identify what conditions you may have in addition to migraine headaches. Let's explore this topic through the lives of the women we met earlier in the book.

Premenstrual Syndrome, Premenstrual Dysphoric Disorder, and Migraine

Beth suffers from PMDD. Premenstrual dysphoric disorder is a more severe form of premenstrual syndrome (PMS), one that involves major emotional ups and downs (mood swings) in addition to the physical symptoms of PMS, such as breast tenderness and bloating, to meet the diagnosis.

Premenstrual syndrome affects 30–80% of women. Physical symptoms include breast tenderness, bloating, joint swelling and joint pain, and emotional symptoms such as depression, anxiety, and irritability. To meet the definition of PMS, there must be a symptom-free period of several weeks after menstruation. Many women think they have PMS when what they have is an underlying mood disorder, such as depression or anxiety, that worsens during the 5-day period before menses and continues into menses. Women should feel 100% free of all PMS symptoms within several days of menstruation; if not, an underlying condition, physical or emotional, should be considered. Premenstrual disorder is strongly associated with migraine. According to several studies, women migraine sufferers may be more likely to suffer from PMS than the general female population.[1,2]

Premenstrual dysphoric disorder is considered a specific mood disorder, and it requires major emotional changes in a woman, such as moderate-severe depression and/or moderate-severe anxiety. In general, it interferes with a woman's ability to function to a greater degree than does PMS. Also, by definition, a woman with PMDD should feel much better within 1 2 days of her period.[3] Only 2–9% of women have PMDD.[4] Medications approved by the U.S. Food and Drug Administration (FDA) for PMDD include Zoloft (sertraline), Sarafem (fluoxetine; also known as Prozac), and Yaz (drospirenone/ethinyl estradiol), an oral birth control pill.

Beth states that she feels fine most of the month but 1–3 days before her period she feels very unstable emotionally. She cries easily, is very irritable, and yells at her boyfriend and family about "little things" that go wrong in her life. She feels like she is "on edge" and ready to explode and lash out at everyone and everything around her. Recently, she got so upset that she threw papers all over her room and screamed so loudly that friends in adjacent dorm rooms came to find out what was wrong. She could not stop screaming and was crying uncontrollably. When her period started the next day, she felt better but was embarrassed by her outbursts the day before. Charting her symptoms over 3 months showed a definite pattern, with emotional instability and outbursts occurring 1–3 days before her period and then feeling better once her period started. She was diagnosed with PMDD and put on Zoloft (sertraline), at 50 mg/day. The Zoloft helped, but Beth found better relief of her symptoms when her doctor upped the dose to 75 mg several days before her period. After her period, she did fine with the 50-mg dose. Beth reports that she still gets migraine that requires a triptan, a migraine-specific medication, despite the Zoloft. She was hoping the Zoloft would prevent the menstrual migraines. However, with the Zoloft, she feels much more "even" emotionally.

Anxiety and Migraine

Lisa, the school teacher with anxiety in addition to her menstrual migraines, reports symptoms such as feeling unable to relax, frequent worry, disturbed sleep, and muscle tension in her neck and upper back.

Her primary care provider recently diagnosed her with generalized anxiety disorder (GAD) and recommended Lexapro (escitalopram).

To find out if you have GAD, like Lisa, ask yourself the following questions:

- Have you had excessive anxiety and worry for longer than 6 months?
- If yes, do you have at least three additional symptoms from the following list?
  - Restlessness
  - Easy fatigue
  - Difficulty concentrating
  - Irritability
  - Muscle tension
  - Disturbed sleep

Anxiety disorders, including GAD, have been associated with migraine. In one study, 9.1% of individuals with migraine had GAD, compared to 2.5% of individuals without migraine.[5] Generalized anxiety disorder is also the most common anxiety disorder seen in primary care. Women are two to three times more at risk for GAD than men; risk increases around the age of 35–45, which is also when migraine prevalence is high.

Other related anxiety disorders such as panic attacks, social phobia, and obsessive-compulsive disorder are higher in migraine sufferers than in the general population.[6] In a study of more than 50,000 adults aged 20 and older, individuals with migraine headache were more likely to have anxiety disorders than the nonheadache control group. In addition, the prevalence of anxiety disorders increased with the number of headache days per month, with those having 15 or more migraine days a month also having the highest rate of anxiety.[7]

Endometriosis and Migraine

Lisa also has been diagnosed with endometriosis, which she knows is linked to infertility. She is concerned because she wants to get pregnant and start a family. However, she has disabling menstrual migraines and is worried about the possible effects of migraine medications in pregnancy. Endometriosis is fairly common in the general population, with a prevalence rate of about 10% in women of child-bearing age. An increased frequency of migraine in women with endometriosis has been documented. In a study of 133 women with endometriosis, 33.8% suffered from migraine, compared to only 15.1% in the control group suffering from migraine.[8] Other studies support this association between migraine and endometriosis. In addition, one study showed that women migraine sufferers with endometriosis have more frequent and disabling headaches than do women without endometriosis who have migraine.[9]

Endometriosis is characterized by pelvic pain and severe menstrual cramps. In endometriosis, pockets of endometrial tissue, similar to the lining of the uterus, are scattered throughout the pelvic area and sometimes into the upper abdomen. This tissue does not show up on pelvic ultrasound. When endometriosis is suspected, a surgical procedure, such as a laparoscopy, is often necessary to diagnose and treat the condition. Laser treatment is often done at the time of surgery to get rid of the endometrial tissue. Medical treatment may include continuous birth control pills and hormone injections, such as Depo-Lupron (leuprolide acetate), to shut down the ovaries; this is often referred to as a "medical oophorectomy" (*oophorectomy* means removal of the ovaries). Pregnancy also can help endometriosis.

Irritable Bowel Syndrome and Migraine

Nancy, the hard-working, driven attorney, suffers from frequent abdominal pain and cramping, often after eating and worse with stress. At times, she has diarrhea; at other times, she has constipation, and she often suffers with gas and bloating. Her diagnosis is irritable bowel syndrome (IBS). She wonders if this diagnosis is related to her migraines.

A large study demonstrated that individuals with IBS have a 60% higher risk of migraine compared to a control group.[10] The common link, researchers believe, may be serotonin, as it is involved in both migraine and the regulation of the digestive tract.

Treatment of IBS usually involves a trial of milk and dairy elimination to see if lactose intolerance is present. A diet rich in fiber can be helpful, and medications for cramping may be needed. On occasion, a selective serotonin reuptake inhibitor like Zoloft (sertraline) is prescribed. Stress reduction is helpful. In my experience, many IBS sufferers are individuals prone to stress.

Abuse and Migraine

In addition to IBS, Nancy has been diagnosed with chronic migraine and medication overuse headache. Her history of episodic migraines, averaging once a week, have transformed or "evolved" into the almost daily headaches she now experiences. Significantly, she suffered from sexual abuse when she was growing up. She suppressed all memories for many years but is now struggling with memories emerging in her dreams, and she's working with a therapist. She asks, "Why should I go to therapy and discuss painful memories? Will therapy help my frequent migraine headaches?"

The lifetime prevalence of physical, sexual, and/or emotional abuse in the general population is 25%, whereas the prevalence of sexual abuse in women with chronic headache is as high as 39–45%.[11] If sexual abuse occurred during childhood, there is a greater risk of headache than if the abuse first occurred in adulthood.[12]

I was an investigator in a multicenter study looking at abuse in women migraine patients. Patients were asked to complete a series of questions (the results were kept confidential). After completing the survey, one of my patients said she wanted to share something that she had never told me before. She went on to admit that when she was growing up, her brother abused her sexually. She had never told me this before out of embarrassment and shame. This experience made me realize that I normally don't ask patients about past history of abuse. It is not a comfortable subject to discuss and is one not often brought up. I encourage you to bring up any past or current issues of abuse, whether physical, emotional, or sexual. As uncomfortable as the discussion may be, not dealing with the issue of abuse can be very damaging to your health, and it may even play a role in your headaches.

Domestic abuse can also exacerbate a headache situation. Home should be a peaceful place. To walk on eggshells around someone, afraid that you may say or do something that will "set them off," indicates a major problem and should be dealt with. I am not suggesting that everyone in a bad marriage should file for divorce; what I am suggesting is that you look at your marriage and relationships and be aware of subtle or overt, obvious abuse and get the counseling and help you need. Most likely, your headaches and overall health, both physical and emotional, will improve.

Posttraumatic Stress Disorder and Migraine

Nancy is frequently awakened in the night with a feeling of great fear. As a young girl, her father would come into her bedroom in the middle of the night and fondle her. She has been diagnosed as suffering from PTSD. The relative frequency of PTSD is higher in chronic migraine sufferers (42.9%) compared to episodic migraine sufferers (9.4%).[13] This higher frequency was seen even after adjusting for depression, which would be expected to be higher in chronic migraine sufferers.

Posttraumatic stress disorder can occur years after abuse, as in Nancy's case; it can occur after a car accident, a fire, a burglary, or any major traumatic event. It is frequently seen in soldiers returning from battle. A combination of therapy and medication is often needed to treat PTSD.

Depression and Migraine

Melanie, the 35-year-old stay-at-home mom, has been feeling depressed and hopeless about her future. Lately, she has turned down invitations to go out with her girlfriends to dinner and a movie, even though her husband has offered to baby-sit. She has lost interest in doing things she used to enjoy, like gardening and playing the piano.

The annual prevalence of depressive disorders is 9.5% in the adult U.S. population. Twice as many women (12%) as men (6%) are affected by a depressive disorder each year. Depressive disorders can include major depressive disorder, dysthymia (a milder form of depression), and bipolar disorder. Looking at major depressive disorder, 6.5% of women suffer from major depressive disorder every year, compared to 3.3% of men.[14] Of migraine sufferers, 17.8% were shown to have a major depressive disorder; those with transformed migraine (also known as chronic migraine) had a 30.3% prevalence.[15] Therefore, migraine itself carries a higher risk of major depressive disorder than that seen in the general population, and those with more frequent migraine have an even higher risk.

Interestingly, a bidirectional influence between depression and migraine has been shown in a large published study. This means that each condition influences the other in a larger than expected way, compared to the general population. In this study, individuals with baseline depression had an increased risk of developing migraine (but not other headaches) over a 2-year period. Meanwhile, those individuals with baseline migraine had an increased risk of developing depression, compared to those with other types of headaches at baseline.[16]

Melanie was diagnosed with major depressive disorder. How do you know if you are suffering from major depressive disorder? Ask yourself the following:

- Have you been feeling depressed every day for 2 weeks or longer?

- Have you lost interest in activities of daily life, including those you used to enjoy, for 2 weeks or longer?

If you answered "yes" to the first two questions, do you suffer from at least three of the following symptoms?

- Weight loss or weight gain
- Over- or undersleeping
- Feeling agitated or slow
- Fatigued or loss of energy
- Feeling worthless or full of guilt
- Difficulty concentrating
- Suicidal thoughts

(This list of symptoms is adapted from a recognized screen for major depressive disorder called the Patient Health Questionnaire-9.)

Anyone can have a "bad day" and feel depressed; that is part of the human condition. But to meet the diagnosis of major depressive disorder, the symptoms of depression need to be present every day for 2 weeks or more.

Bipolar disorder falls under the general category of depressive disorders. It is characterized by mood swings, including episodes of mania or hypomania, and it affects 2.3 million adult Americans, with equal prevalence in men and women. Individuals with bipolar disorder are more likely to suffer from migraine than are the general population. In a published study of 37,000 individuals, women with bipolar disorder showed a 34.7% incidence of migraine, in contrast to only 14.7% migraine in women without bipolar disorder.[17] If you wonder if you have bipolar disorder, discuss your concerns with your medical provider. Bipolar disorder often runs in families. To learn more, go to www.nami.org.

Many antidepressants and some of the mood stabilizers used to treat bipolar disorder may be effective for migraine prevention as well. It is always important to monitor your headaches, including menstrual migraine, when medications for other medical conditions are prescribed. Many sure your headache doctor is aware of all the medications you are taking.

Fibromyalgia and Migraine

In addition to depression, Melanie is experiencing a persistent feeling of fatigue and pain all over her body, especially in her neck and upper back. A physician she saw suggested that she may be suffering from *fibromyalgia*. Fibromyalgia is a chronic pain syndrome characterized by pain all over the body that lasts for more than 3 months. Extreme tenderness in certain muscle spots is often present. Fibromyalgia is present in 2% of the population, with women having a 3.4% prevalence, compared to 0.5% of men.[18]

There is a strong connection between fibromyalgia and headache, with 50% of fibromyalgia patients reporting headache. In a study of migraine patients, 22% had fibromyalgia, compared to 2% of the general population.[19] In a study of fibromyalgia patients, 76% reported headache, and 63% of these had migraine.[20] There appears to be a strong association between migraine and fibromyalgia, pointing to a shared underlying mechanism. In both conditions, individuals exhibit a high sensitivity to their environment, as compared to the general population.

In my experience, most fibromyalgia patients have some degree of depression. It is not uncommon for patients in my practice to suffer from menstrual migraine, fibromyalgia, and depression. As a general practitioner, I need to look at the "whole person," with all medical conditions integrated, in order to best manage an individual's migraines.

Current FDA-approved medications for fibromyalgia include Cymbalta (duloxetine), Savella (milnacipran), and Lyrica (pregabalin). Cymbalta is also FDA approved for depression; Lyrica is FDA approved for shingles (herpes zoster) and peripheral neuropathy. Patients with fibromyalgia are often put on several daily medications that work together to help their pain. I have used all three of these FDA-approved medications with my patients who have fibromyalgia and migraines. These medications may help to prevent migraine, even though they are not FDA approved for migraine prevention. Patients with fibromyalgia appear to be especially sensitive to medications, so it is important to start with a very low dose of any medication and gradually increase the dose.

Other treatments for fibromyalgia may include massage therapy, acupuncture, physical therapy, stress-reduction training, trigger point injections, and numerous other treatments. Tricyclic antidepressants such as Elavil (amitriptyline) and Pamelor (nortriptyline) are often used to help lessen chronic muscle pain and to help with sleep. This class of medication may help prevent migraine as well. Energizing antidepressants such as Prozac (fluoxetine) are often used in the morning to help treat fatigue. Muscle relaxants can be used but have the troublesome side-effect of sedation and so are best taken at night.

Sleep Disorders and Migraine

Theresa, 40, is going through a messy divorce. She is having a lot of trouble sleeping. She is working with a divorce attorney, and she struggles to be strong emotionally for her sons. Her migraines are increasing in frequency and severity. She approaches her doctor and asks, "Can I have something to help me sleep? Do you think if I get a better night's sleep, my headaches will get better?"

Sleep deprivation, including trouble getting to sleep and trouble staying asleep, is frequently reported in migraine and, in fact, is more commonly reported as a trigger for migraine in women than in men.[21] In addition, women who have chronic migraine have a very high prevalence of poor quality (nonrestorative) sleep. In a study of 147 women with chronic migraine, 83.7% reported feeling tired on awakening. Over half of the women reported difficulty falling asleep.[22] Snoring has also been linked to chronic headache.[23] This association was independent of weight, gender, and age.

To improve her sleep and migraines, Theresa was given a referral for cognitive-behavioral therapy, which has been shown to improve headache frequency and intensity.[24]

I have often prescribed sleeping pills such as Lunesta (eszopiclone) or Ambien (zolpidem) in my patients suffering with insomnia. In some individual cases, I have seen a remarkable reduction in headache simply by restoring a good night's sleep. Melatonin, an over-the-counter sleep aid, can be helpful and now comes in an extended-release (ER) form.

Patients like Theresa are often frustrated when they have a Saturday or Sunday morning headache after sleeping in. Migraine attacks have been associated with oversleeping as well as with undersleeping. Migraine sufferers do best if they establish regular sleeping habits, including going to bed and getting up at the same time every day.

Obesity and Migraine

Obesity has been associated with migraine, especially as a risk factor for the development of chronic daily headache.[25] In a study of 721 migraine patients, anxiety and depression were also associated with obesity. Increasing obesity as measured by body mass risk was associated with worsening migraine attack severity and frequency.[26] But the association between migraine and obesity in migraine individuals who do not have mood disorders has not been clearly defined.

Obesity is also linked to snoring and sleep disorders, such as sleep apnea, which can aggravate migraines. Exercise, good eating habits, and maintaining a normal body weight is recommended for all migraine patients.

Stroke Risk and Migraine

Forty-seven-year old Christy is going through perimenopause and experiencing an increase in her headaches. She is thinking about going on estrogen for her symptoms but is very concerned about the risk of stroke since she read that estrogen increases stroke risk, especially in someone with migraine headaches.

Kate, the 55-year-old woman with a history of menstrual migraines, is now suffering from severe menopausal symptoms. Although interested in the benefits of estrogen, she is worried about stroke risk.

The risk of stroke in migraine has been well-documented in numerous studies. The risk of stroke is greater in migraine with aura compared to migraine without aura.[27] However, even young women without aura have a higher risk of stroke than do young women without migraine. The absolute risk is low but increases with smoking and the use of estrogen-containing birth control pills.[28] The risk of stroke also increases with obesity and uncontrolled high blood pressure. Any history of a clotting disorder in an individual or her family will raise particular concern about the risk of stroke in a migraine patient. The decision of whether an individual female migraine patient can be safely put on an estrogen-containing birth control pill depends on many factors. We will explore this issue in detail in Chapter 6.

A very large study published in 2005 showed a 1.7% increase in stroke risk in women migraine patients who reported visual aura with their migraine attacks, but no increase in stroke risk in women without visual aura symptoms. For older women like Christy and Kate, the data are reassuring. In this study, the risk of stroke was highest in women aged 45–55 years, but this risk was not seen in older women.[29]

Therefore, it is very important to have your migraine attacks clearly diagnosed as with or without aura. If you suffer from migraines without aura (as is true for the majority of women migraine sufferers), your risk of stroke is very low, comparable to that of the general population. Most women like Christy and Kate can treat their hot flashes and night sweats with estrogen without significantly increasing their stroke risk. For more information on deciding if hormone therapy right for you, refer to Chapter 6.

Occasionally, the issue of patent foramen ovale is raised by a female migraine patient in my practice. *Patent foramen ovale* refers to an opening between the upper chambers of the heart (the right and left atrium). In the more severe cases, there can be "shunting" of the blood, in that less-oxygenated blood gets shunted into the left upper chamber and then pumped out to the rest of the body. Patent foramen ovale has been linked to young stroke patients with migraine, especially migraine with aura. However, patent foramen ovale is found in as much as 10% of the general population. A few years ago, a clinical trial was done to see if closing the patent foramen ovale would reduce migraine frequency. In this study, 42% of the patients had at least a 50% reduction in migraine days compared to only 23% of patients in the sham (placebo) arm of the study.[30] However, there are risks with this surgical procedure. Currently, the benefits do not seem to outweigh the risks of undergoing this procedure in the majority of migraine patients with patent foramen ovale.

Conclusion

As we've seen in this chapter, many migraine sufferers have medical conditions in addition to their migraine headaches. Many medical conditions, such as depression, fibromyalgia, anxiety, and history of abuse, are more common in women migraine sufferers than in the general population. Being aware of all your medical conditions is critical to developing an effective management plan for your migraines, including menstrual migraines. I hope this chapter has helped you take a thorough inventory of all your symptoms and conditions. If you are not sure if you are suffering from some of the conditions described in this chapter, I encourage you to see your doctor and get properly diagnosed.

References

1. Keenan PA, Lindamer LA. Non-migraine headache across the menstrual cycle in women with and without premenstrual syndrome. Cephalalgia. 1992; 12: 356–359.

2. Keenan PA. Migraine and premenstrual syndrome. Cephalalgia. 1993; 13: 377.

3. American Psychiatric Association. *Diagnostic and Statistical Manual of Mental Disorders*, Fourth Edition (DSM-IV). Washington, DC: American Psychiatric Association; 1994.

4. Yonkers KA. Antidepressants in the treatment of premenstrual dysphoric disorder. J Clin Psychiatry. 1997; 58(suppl 14): 4–13.

5. McWilliams L, Goodwin RD, Cox BJ. Depression and anxiety associated with three pain conditions: results from a nationally representative sample. Pain. 2004; 111(1–2); 77–83.

6. Merikangas KR, Stevens DE. Comorbidity of migraine and psychiatric disorders. Neurol Clin. 1997; 15: 115–123.

7. Zwart JA, Dyb G, Hagen K, et al. Depression and anxiety disorders associated with headache frequency. The Nord-Trondelag Health Study. Eur J Neurol. 2003; 10(2): 147–152.

8. Ferrero S, Pretta S, Bertoldi S, et al. Increased frequency of migraine among women with endometriosis. Hum Reprod. 2004; 19: 2927–2932.

9. Tietjen GE, Bushnell CD, Herial NA, et al. Endometriosis is associated with prevalence of comorbid conditions in migraine. Headache. 2007; 47: 1069–1078.

10. Cole J, Rothman KJ, Cabral HJ, et al. Migraine, fibromyalgia and depression among people with IBS: A prevalence study. Brit Med Coun Gastroenterol. 2006; 6: 26–30.

11. Nelson HD, Nygren P, McInerney Y, et al. Screening women and elderly adults for family and intimate partner violence: a review of the evidence for the US Preventive Services Task Force. Ann Intern Med. 2004; 140: 387–396.

12. Golding JM. Sexual assault history and headache: five population studies. J Nerv Ment Dis. 1999; 187: 624–629.

13. Peterlin BL, Tietjen G, Meng S, et al. Post-traumatic stress disorder in episodic and chronic migraine. Headache. 2008; 48: 517–522.

14. National Institute of Mental Health. The numbers count: mental disorders in America, depressive disorders. 2001, www.nimh.nih.gov/publicat/numbers.cf

15. Buse D, et al. Results of the American Migraine Prevalence and Prevention (AMPP) study: comorbidity of depression, obesity, disability and headache. Poster presented at AAN Annual Meeting Boston, MA, 2007.

16. Breslau N, Lipton RB, Stewart WF, et al. Comorbidity of migraine and depression: investigating potential etiology and prognosis. Neurology. 2003; 60: 1308–1312.

17. McIntyre RS, Konarski JZ, Wilkins K, et al. The prevalence and impact of migraine headache in bipolar disorder: results from the Canadian Community Health Survey. Headache. 2006; 46: 973–982.

18. Abeles AM, Pillinger MH, Solitar BM, et al. Narrative review: the pathophysiology of fibromyalgia. Ann Intern Med. 2007: 146: 726–734.

19. Ifergane G, Buskila D, Simiseshvely N, et al. Prevalence of fibromyalgia syndrome in migraine patients. Cephalalgia. 2005; 26: 451–456.

20. Marcus DA, Bernstein C, Rudy TE. Fibromyalgia and headache: an epidemiological study supporting migraine as part of the fibromyalgia syndrome. Clin Rheumatol. 2005; 24: 595–601.

21. Rasmussen BK. Migraine and tension type headache in a general population: precipitating factors, female hormones, sleep pattern and relation to lifestyle. Pain. 1993; 53: 65–72.

22. Calhoun AH, Ford S, Finkel AG, et al. The prevalence and spectrum of sleep problems in women with transformed migraine. Headache. 2006; 46: 604–610.

23. Scher A, Lipton RB, Stewart WF. Habitual snoring as a risk factor for chronic daily headache. Neurology. 2003; 60: 1366–1368.

24. Calhoun AH, Ford S. Behavioral sleep modification may revert transformed migraine to episodic migraine. Headache. 2007; 47: 1178–1184.

25. Scher A, Stewart WF, Ricci JA, et al. Factors associated with the onset and remission of chronic daily headache in a population-based study. Pain. 2003; 1061: 81 89.

26. Tietjen GE, Peterlin BL, Brandes JL, et al. Depression and anxiety: effect on the migraine-obesity relationship. Headache. 2007; 47(6): 866–875.

27. Rothrock J, North J, Madden K, et al. Migraine and migrainous stroke: risk factors and prognosis. Neurology. 1993; 43: 2473–2476.

28. Tzourio C, Kittner SJ, Bousser MG, et al. Migraine and stroke in young women. Cephalalgia. 2000; 20: 190–199.

29. Kurth T, Slomke MA, Kase CS, et al. Migraine, headache, and the risk of stroke in women: a prospective study. Neurology. 2005; 64: 1573–1577.

30. Tepper SJ, Sheftell FD, Bigal ME. The patent foramen ovale-migraine question. Neuro Sci. 28(suppl): S118–S123.

5

Treatment

TREATMENT OF MIGRAINE HEADACHES, INCLUDING menstrual-related migraines, can be divided into acute, preventive, and "mini" or short-term preventive treatment. In this chapter, we discuss each type of treatment in detail and lay out reasonable expectations for each. We include over-the-counter and herbal treatment. Keep in mind that no one treatment will work for all women suffering with migraine. Also, a treatment plan that works for a while may stop working after a period of time. In those cases, a new treatment plan may need to be developed. The dosing information and specific treatments described in this chapter are for educational purposes only. Readers should talk to their healthcare providers to get the best care for their individual needs.

BOX 5-1 ONE AND DONE

Many of my patients wonder if it is reasonable to hope for an acute migraine treatment that will work completely in a single dose. A colleague of mine coined the phrase "one and done"

(continued)

> **BOX 5-1 (Continued)**
>
> to capture this sought-after treatment. There is good news for migraine sufferers: You should absolutely seek a "one and done" treatment for acute migraine. It is a reasonable goal, and you deserve it!

Acute Migraine Treatment

Acute treatment is intended to take care of the current problem—the headache that is present. A reasonable goal for a migraine attack is to find a treatment that will take away the headache completely in 2 hours. Ideally, the treatment will be well-tolerated and have little to no side effects. An additional goal would be for all the associated migraine symptoms—like nausea and vomiting, sensitivity to light and noise, neck pain, and sinus symptoms such as facial pain and nasal congestion—to go away. A return to full function—whether that is at work or home—is a reasonable expectation for most acute treatments. Last, the headache should stay away once it has gone away. Thus, the right acute treatment should:

- Take the headache pain away completely in 2 hours
- Take away all associated migraine symptoms, such as nausea
- Keep the headache pain away for at least 24 hours
- Be powerful enough to work in one dose, without the need for any additional medication in most cases (sometimes this is not possible)

Acute treatment is taken when and *only* when the migraine attack is occurring. Ideally, acute treatment is not needed more than twice a week, unless the problem is a menstrual migraine or prolonged migraine attack. Many women in my practice take acute medication for 3–5 days in a row for their menstrual migraines but rarely need acute treatment more than once or twice a week during the nonmenstrual times of their cycle.

Why is it so important to limit acute treatment?

The main reason is to prevent *medication overuse* or *rebound* headaches. This is a condition in which the body and brain get so acclimated to a medication that tolerance is developed and a headache will occur unless the medication is taken. A common example of this in everyday life is the effect that caffeine has on many of us. The caffeine included in Excedrin (an acetaminophen-aspirin-caffeine combination) is partly responsible for the big problem that I see in my practice with daily rebound headaches. I have taken the headache history of many patients who share a similar story:

Nancy tells me she is having a daily low-grade headache in addition to her more severe, disabling menstrual migraines. She is quick to point out that her daily headaches are not migraine. I ask Nancy what she takes for her daily headaches. Not surprisingly, she tells me that she takes Excedrin, anywhere from six to twelve tablets a day. The Excedrin helps, briefly, but then the headache comes back, and she reacts by taking another dose.

Many women find themselves on this same roller coaster. Often, the overused medication is a prescription, like Vicodin (hydrocodone), Fiorinal (butalbital-aspirin-caffeine combination), or Fioricet (butalbital-acetaminophen-caffeine), or even a triptan like Imitrex (sumatriptan). In most cases, the medication is appropriate and makes sense when it is initially chosen as the acute medication for migraine attacks. Unfortunately, over time, use of the medication escalates, and the very medication that a person takes for her headache becomes the cause of the now almost-daily headache. To prevent this rebound headache pattern, it is important not to take acute medication too often. Ideally, acute medication for migraine attacks is not taken more than twice a week.

Types of Acute Medication

Acute medication can be divided into migraine-specific and migraine-nonspecific medication. Migraine-specific medications target the migraine pain pathway and are used in acute situations. Generally, these are medications primarily indicated for migraine headaches. Examples include the ergots, ergot alkaloids, and triptans (these will be explained in more detail later in this chapter). Nonspecific acute migraine medications include over-the-counter medications like Excedrin, Advil (ibuprofen), Aleve (naproxen), aspirin, and Tylenol (acetaminophen), and a wide variety of prescription medications like Fiorinal (butalbital-aspirin-caffeine), Fioricet (butalbital-acetaminophen-caffeine), Vicodin (hydrocodone), Midrin (isometheptene mucate-dichloralphenazone-acetaminophen combination), codeine, muscle relaxants, and antiemetic (antivomiting/nausea) medications such as Compazine (prochlorperazine), Phenergan (promethazine), Reglan (metoproclamide), and Zofran (ondansetron). In addition, acute medications can be divided by formulation (the type of medication in terms of oral or nonoral administration, such as injections or nasal sprays).

In picking the best acute medication for migraine attacks, it is important to assess the severity of the migraine attacks and to identify the associated symptoms, such as nausea or vomiting. If there is significant nausea or vomiting, a nonoral medication should be chosen. If the headache rapidly escalates or builds to severe pain, then a medication delivered via injection may be better since nonoral medications, especially injections, can kick in and take effect within 10 minutes. We'll explore all the options in greater detail in the upcoming sections. As you read the next section, ask yourself the following questions:

- Do I usually have nausea and/or vomiting with my migraine attacks?
- Do my headaches rapidly escalate from mild to severe?
- Do I wake up with morning migraines that are moderate to severe?
- Am I satisfied with my current treatment?
- Am I completely headache free and back to full function in 2 hours?
- Do I ever have to re-dose my medication?
- Do I have to have a "rescue" or second medication for the headache?

- Do I have any side effects from my current acute migraine medication?

If you answered "yes" to one or more of these questions, it is possible that you may benefit from a change in your acute migraine medication treatment, including that taken for menstrual migraine. Read on.

Over-the-Counter Treatments

Acetaminophen

Acetaminophen (as is found in the brand name medication Tylenol) is an over-the-counter analgesic (pain reliever) that is approved for use for the relief of minor aches, pain, and fever. It has been available as a nonprescription medication for more than 50 years. It is often found in combination with other analgesics, such as aspirin, and with prescription pain medications, such as Fioricet (butalbital-acetaminophen-caffeine) and Vicodin (hydrocodone). It does not tend to irritate the stomach like aspirin does. For individuals who have ulcer or stomach issues, acetaminophen may be a better choice than aspirin. Also, acetaminophen is often the preferred headache medication in pregnancy or in women trying to get pregnant. The treatment goal is to be headache free and back to full function in 2 hours.

> Dose: 1,000 mg every 4–6 hours, to a maximum of 4 g/day
> Warning: Can affect the liver. Do not use if liver problems are present.

Is Acetaminophen Effective for the Acute Treatment of a Migraine Attack?

In a recent study published in the journal *Headache* (May 2010), acetaminophen at a dose of 1,000 mg was shown to be an effective and well-tolerated treatment for episodic and moderate migraine headache.[1] In addition, acetaminophen provided a beneficial effect on the associated symptoms of migraine, including nausea, photophobia (sensitivity to light), phonophobia (sensitivity to noise), and functional disability (interference with ability to function with daily activities of living). There were 346 patients enrolled and treated in this study, conducted at 13 primary care sites in the United States. Each patient was randomly assigned to a single 1,000 mg dose of acetaminophen or placebo. Placebo is a treatment given to "mimic" the active treatment being given; placebo treatment would not contain any of the active ingredient. This was a double-blind clinical trial, so neither the investigators nor the subjects knew which medication they were given. Of the 346 subjects, 177 received the acetaminophen and 160 received the placebo.

Significantly, more patients treated with the acetaminophen (52%) reported mild to no pain after 2 hours compared with those treated with placebo (32%). An improvement in migraine-associated symptoms such as nausea and sensitivity to light was stronger in the acetaminophen group compared to placebo. No serious adverse events or side effects were noted in either group.

Box 5-2

Acetaminophen at a dose of 1,000 mg is inexpensive, well-tolerated, and may be an effective treatment for mild to moderate migraine attacks. It may help some of the associated symptoms of migraine including nausea, sensitivity to light and noise, and disability. It is generally considered safe during pregnancy. However, for more moderate to severe migraine attacks, acetaminophen is unlikely to meet our treatment goal of being headache free and back to full function in 2 hours, especially when dealing with menstrual migraine!

Aspirin (Salicylate)

Aspirin is an over-the-counter analgesic for pain and fever. It has anti inflammatory activity that acetaminophen does not have, and it may be more effective for acute migraine attacks than acetaminophen. However, it can upset the stomach and increase the risk of ulcers, aggravate bleeding disorders, and cause kidney damage in some individuals. It is often taken in combination with other medications, such as acetaminophen and caffeine (via Excedrin) or with butalbital and caffeine (Fiorinal). The treatment goal is the same: headache free and back to full function in 2 hours. If aspirin can achieve this goal and is not taken more than twice a week, then it may be an appropriate acute migraine medication for some migraine attacks in some individuals. For most pregnant patients, however, aspirin-containing products should be avoided primarily because of the bleeding risk.

> Dose: 325–650 mg every 4–6 hours, to a maximum of 4 g/day
> Warning: Can cause gastrointestinal upset or bleeding; kidney problems can occur if taken in excess.

Aspirin is most commonly used for migraine in a combination product known as Excedrin. Excedrin (also marketed as Excedrin Migraine) contains acetaminophen and caffeine in addition to aspirin. In clinical trials assessing the effectiveness of this combination as acute treatment of mild to moderate migraine, pain relief was significantly greater in migraine individuals taking the combination product compared to those taking placebo.[2]

The delivery system of a medication can make a difference in its effectiveness. In a published study comparing an effervescent form of aspirin (meaning it bubbles and breaks apart quickly when put into water or swallowed) with Imitrex (sumatriptan) at 50 mg and ibuprofen at 400 mg, the effervescent aspirin was as effective as the sumatriptan (50 mg) or the ibuprofen (400 mg) as an acute therapy for migraine.[3] This is a result that would not be expected with aspirin in its regular tablet form.

> **Box 5-3**
>
> Aspirin may be effective for mild to moderate migraine attack. It may be more effective if taken as a combination product, as in Excedrin (acetaminophen-aspirin-caffeine), or if taken in an effervescent form that dissolves quickly. Aspirin is best avoided if a woman is pregnant or if there are significant gastrointestinal issues, such as an ulcer, or bleeding disorders.

Caffeine

Caffeine is often used for migraine attacks, either as a single agent or in combination with simple analgesics such as acetaminophen and aspirin, or with prescription medications such as butalbital (Fiorinal, Fioricet). Caffeine acts as a vasoconstrictor in that it can constrict (make smaller) the throbbing blood vessels that are often part of a migraine attack. If a person does not normally drink a lot of caffeine, then having a cup of coffee or a cola soft drink can be quite helpful in treating a migraine. I was once stuck at an airport with a throbbing headache and nausea and without any of my usual migraine medications. I sipped coffee, alternating with water and an antacid (Mylanta), and gradually the migraine lessened. However, if a person drinks a lot of caffeine on a daily basis, her body and blood vessels will be accustomed to caffeine and it may not work as well for an acute migraine attack.

A note about kids: Some of my pediatric patients will split a Coke with Mom when migraines occur, and it works well! In these cases, the child is not normally allowed to drink caffeine so, if taken only when a headache is present, the caffeine can work well to relieve the attack. I have also seen a beneficial effect in pregnant women who may have given up their daily caffeine. Since they are not ingesting caffeine on a daily basis (although most obstetricians allow their pregnant patients to have caffeine in moderation), it can be very helpful when taken for an acute migraine attack during pregnancy.

Box 5-4

Caution: Caffeine can often lead to rebound headaches, so be careful. Some of my patients have reported great improvement in their headaches if they give up caffeine. But it doesn't work for everyone. I tried to stop caffeine but found myself irritable and missing my morning coffee. My advice for most migraine patients is to keep their caffeine intake in moderation. For most of us, moderation is to limit our caffeinated beverages to two servings a day, whether it is coffee, tea, or cola.

Combination Simple Analgesics

Over-the-counter combination products usually contain two or three of either acetaminophen, aspirin, or caffeine. The most commonly used combination product for acute migraine attacks that I see in my practice is Excedrin (acetaminophen-aspirin-caffeine) and, as discussed earlier, it is widely known for causing medication overuse headache or what is commonly referred to as "rebound headache." My advice: Limit Excedrin to a maximum of two doses a week. It is an appropriate acute migraine medication if it helps you meet your treatment goals, but if you find yourself taking it more than twice a week, ask your healthcare provider to find a different medication to treat your acute migraine attacks.

Excedrin is the first nonprescription medication to be approved by the U.S. Food and Drug Administration (FDA) to treat migraine. Excedrin is marketed for many conditions and is also sold under the label Excedrin Migraine. The ingredients are identical to regular Excedrin.

Sadly, by the time many patients come into my practice, they are taking Excedrin daily and don't know how to stop the vicious cycle. If they don't take it, their headaches worsen; but, even with treatment, they need to keep taking it and often their headaches never lessen to "zero." In other words, many are simply dulling their headache; they are in such a terrible rebound cycle that their headaches are daily and all the Excedrin is doing, at best, is providing temporary relief.

> **BOX 5-5**
>
> *Never get in the habit of taking acute migraine medication more than twice a week on average.* The only exception may be during the week of menstrual migraine, when acute medication is needed daily. In my opinion, this treatment approach is all right as long as you only use acute medication daily during the menstrual migraine period.

In Germany, a popular over-the-counter combination medication is used that contains acetylsalicylic acid (aspirin), paracetamol (similar to acetaminophen), and caffeine. In a large clinical trial of 1,743 patients, pain reduction was greater in the group taking the combination product than in those taking a single agent, such as aspirin or paracetamol.[4] It appears that combination products may be more effective than single-medication products for some migraine attacks.

Antinausea Medications

Over-the-counter antinausea medications may be useful for the nausea and vomiting that are often part of the acute migraine attack. However, prescription strength antinausea medications are generally more effective for acute migraine than are over-the-counter products and will be discussed in more detail later in this chapter. Mylanta, Maalox, and Pepto-Bismol are easily accessible medications that may be somewhat helpful for the gastrointestinal symptoms often accompanying migraine.

Nonsteroidal Anti-Inflammatory Products (NSAIDs)

This group of acute medications includes aspirin, ibuprofen (Motrin, Advil), naproxen (Naprosyn), and naproxen sodium (Aleve, Anaprox). The NSAID class of medications is widely available in over-the-counter dosages, as well as in prescription-strength dosages. Most migraine studies have been conducted using prescription-strength NSAID products. A recent review of naproxen sodium in 16 clinical trials for the acute treatment of migraine concluded that naproxen is more effective than placebo but may cause more side effects, such as nausea, dizziness, gastrointestinal upset, and abdominal pain.[5] The dosage used in the studies ranged from 500 to 825 mg. In the United States, 220–550 mg is the dosage range for a single dose of naproxen sodium, and this dose can be repeated after 12 hours. Thus, the normal daily recommended dose should not exceed 1,100 mg. Anaprox, a prescription drug, is available as a 275 mg tablet and Anaprox DS (DS = double strength) as a 550 mg tablet. Naproxen sodium at prescription strength relieves pain faster and is the preferred agent. Over-the-counter Aleve is naproxen sodium and comes as a 220 mg tablet; I allow my patients to take two at a time, which is close to the prescription strength.

Naprosyn (naproxen) comes in 250, 375, 500 mg tablets and as a 125 mg per teaspoon suspension (liquid). It can be helpful, but it is not as quick-acting as the naproxen sodium products Aleve and Anaprox.

Recommendations for Use of Naproxen

- The preferred choice is the naproxen sodium form (Aleve, Anaprox) of naproxen because it is absorbed faster and, accordingly, relieves pain faster than naproxen by itself.
- A higher dose should be used at the onset of the headache (e.g., two Aleve or one Anaprox DS; and repeat dose in 12 hours if necessary).
- It's okay to keep taking the dose every 12 hours until you are free from headache and back to full function.

- Take with food to prevent gastrointestinal upset. Naproxen may be taken with other migraine medications, such as a triptan, to increase effectiveness (see the triptan section in this chapter).
- Do not use during pregnancy.
- It's okay to take naproxen while breastfeeding.

Ibuprofen is sold over-the-counter as Motrin and Advil, in both tablet and liquid form. Advil is approved by the FDA for the acute treatment of migraine and is sold as Advil Migraine. The dose for acute migraine can vary from 200 to 800 mg and can be repeated every 4 hours, with a usual maximum dosage of 3,200 mg per day (four dosages of 800 mg). Ibuprofen can be an effective acute migraine medication.

Ibuprofen or Naproxen Sodium: Which Is Better?

Naproxen has a longer half-life and duration of action than does ibuprofen. The half-life of naproxen is between 12 and 15 hours, compared to 2 hours for ibuprofen. Therefore, in some patients, there may be an advantage in staying headache-free for a longer period of time after taking naproxen than ibuprofen.

However, individual experiences vary. The answer is going to be different for different individuals. Whichever one works best for you is the one that is better! Remember, the goal is to be headache free and back to full function in 2 hours. Some migraine patients will achieve this with ibuprofen whereas others will prefer naproxen.

Cambia: A New NSAID

Cambia (diclofenac) is an oral form of diclofenac, an NSAID, and the only NSAID currently approved in the United States for the acute treatment of migraine. The dose is 50 mg for 24 hours. Cambia is packaged as a powder; it is mixed with 1–2 ounces of water and swallowed. It is well-tolerated in clinical studies and has an onset of action that is faster than the tablet form of diclofenac. The time to begin working is 15 minutes. Significantly, it has a low recurrence rate, meaning that once it begins working, it continues to be effective. It can be taken anytime during the migraine attack. It may work better and faster than oral ibuprofen and naproxen for some patients. For many of my patients, Cambia is their preferred NSAID for acute migraine treatment.

Toradol

Toradol (ketorolac) is an NSAID that comes in both an oral tablet and an injectable form. The injection is often given in 30–60 mg dosages and can be very useful in treating an acute migraine attack. It is not addictive like narcotic and opioid medications. Injectable ketorolac is often the preferred medication when patients come to an urgent care facility with a severe migraine. It does not cause drowsiness, so a patient can drive herself to the office, get the injection, and, when better, drive herself home. The injection also can be self-administered with proper instruction. Studies have shown that a migraine attack can progress to the point at which no oral medication can rescue the patient, and it then needs to be treated with a nonoral medication. A ketorolac injection can be very useful in treating severe migraine attacks, including menstrual migraine.

Why Do NSAIDs Work in Migraine Attacks?

Because migraine is an inflammatory event, NSAIDs are effective because their main action is anti-inflammatory. These medications act to prevent the production of *prostaglandins*, pathway chemicals involved in migraine. By inhibiting or preventing prostaglandin production, the migraine pathway is interrupted. NSAIDs work best if taken early in the migraine attack. However, studies now indicate that NSAIDs can still be effective later in the attack, and they may prevent some of the "fogginess" and lack of mental alertness that many patients describe having after the headache goes away.

Acute Medications (Prescription)

Triptans

Let's now turn our attention to prescription medications that are commonly used for the acute treatment of migraine attacks. This section is divided into migraine-specific acute medications and migraine-nonspecific medications. The triptans are the most migraine-specific class of medication we have to treat acute migraine attacks. In 1993, the first triptan was made available in the United States as the Imitrex (sumatriptan) injection. It has revolutionized the treatment of migraine and, in my opinion, is the most significant advance in the treatment of migraine in the past 50 years.

Soon after the introduction of the Imitrex injection into the marketplace, an oral and a nasal spray form of Imitrex became available. We then could tailor the delivery system of Imitrex to the type of migraine attack. For example, if the individual was nauseated and vomiting, a nonoral route of delivery, like the nasal spray or injection, made sense. If the headache was not as severe and there was no vomiting, then the oral tablet might be more convenient. For many migraine patients, Imitrex was a miracle. I will never forget when, right after Imitrex was introduced, a patient said to me, "Dr. Hutchinson, when I look back on the year 1993, the most significant event was finding out that my headaches were migraine and then taking Imitrex. For the first time in years, I had something that would help my headaches."

Box 5-6

Before triptans were available, many of my patients were using nonspecific medications to treat their migraines. For many of them, these medications did not give them complete relief and often caused side effects such as drowsiness. It was common for patients to take narcotics and sedatives for their migraines

(continued)

BOX 5-6   (Continued)

such as Vicodin (hydrocodone) and Fiorinal (butalbital aspirin caffeine) or Fioricet (butalbital-acetaminophen-caffeine). They accepted the fact that they would be "down" for the rest of the day and have to sleep or stay home after taking these medications. With triptans, most patients can take the medication, be headache free in 2 hours; and return to full function!

Seven different triptan medications are available in the United States. They are:

- Amerge (naratriptan)
- Axert (almotriptan)
- Frova (frovatriptan)
- Imitrex (sumatriptan)
- Maxalt (rizatriptan)
- Relpax (eletriptan)
- Zomig (zolmitriptan)

A novel triptan-NSAID combination tablet is also available in the United States. It is called Treximet (sumatriptan-naproxen sodium) and, in my opinion, it is the most migraine-targeted medication available for the acute treatment of migraine. It treats multiple pathways involved in migraine and may be more effective for many individuals than taking a triptan alone.

Let's now discuss each triptan specifically:

- *Amerge (naratriptan)* comes in a 1 mg and 2.5 mg tablet. A second dose can be taken after 4 hours; the maximum daily dose is 5 mg. It is considered a "long-acting" triptan; it may not kick in as quickly as the shorter-acting triptans (Axert, Imitrex, Maxalt, Relpax, and Zomig) but may have fewer side effects in some individuals. It has been well-studied in the prevention of menstrual migraine.

- *Axert (almotriptan)* comes in a 6.25 and 12.5 mg tablet. It can be repeated after 2 hours; the maximum daily dose is 25 mg. It is a short-acting triptan but may not be effective enough for some patients. Many headache specialists have found it to be not as effective as the other short-acting triptans (Imitrex, Maxalt, Relpax, and Zomig), but individual experiences vary. It is the first triptan to be FDA approved for use in the adolescent population. It is very well-tolerated and may have fewer side effects than other oral triptans. A rigorous study concluded that almotriptan is effective and well-tolerated in adolescents aged 12–17.[6]

- *Frova (frovatriptan)* comes in a 2.5 mg tablet. A second dose can be taken after 2 hours; a third dose can be taken 2 hours later, and the maximum daily dose is 7.5 mg. It is considered the longest acting of all the triptans and, in general, its effects lasts for 26 hours. This can be an advantage for long-lasting migraine attacks, such as menstrual migraine. It has been well studied for the prevention of menstrual migraine, and it is well-tolerated by most individuals.

- *Imitrex (sumatriptan)* comes in 25, 50, and 100 mg tablets. It also comes in a 5 mg and a 20 mg nasal spray, and as a 4 mg and 6 mg injection. It was the first triptan available, and it has been shown to be very effective for many migraine patients. The injection and nasal spray forms can be useful for migraine attacks associated with nausea and/or vomiting, as well as for attacks that are rapidly escalating. The injection begins working in 10 minutes for most individuals, and the nasal spray begins working in 15 minutes. The injectable form is considered by many headache specialists to be the best medication we have available to treat acute migraine. The oral Imitrex can be repeated after 2 hours; the maximum daily dose is 200 mg. The 100 mg strength tablet is considered the most effective for most adults. The nasal spray is usually given in the 20 mg strength in adults and may be repeated after 2 hours, with the maximum daily dose of 40 mg or two sprays in 24 hours. For the injection, 4 or 6 mg may be given and then repeated in 1 hour to a maximum of 12 mg in 24 hours. The

Imitrex injection is the only triptan to have FDA approval to treat cluster as well as migraine headache. (See Chapter 3 to read about the difference between a cluster headache and a migraine headache).

- In 2010, a new delivery system for Imitrex injection became available under the name of Sumavel Dose Pro. This unique, needle-free delivery system delivers 6 mg of Imitrex into the subcutaneous tissue of the thigh or abdomen by compressed nitrogen gas. The compressed nitrogen gas is contained in the back chamber of the administration device and, when activated, forces the front chamber to deliver the medication into the tissue. For patients who are afraid of needles or who find the current Imitrex needle delivery system confusing, this new system offers an advantage. A study examining ease of use found that 51 of 52 patients who opened the packaging of at least one of the needle-free systems used it successfully the first time.[7] The effectiveness of this needle-free system is expected to be the same as the needle injection, because it delivers the same medication. Like the Imitrex needle delivery system, the Sumavel Dose Pro can be repeated after 1 hour to a maximum of two doses or 12 mg in 24 hours.

Who is a good candidate for Imitrex injectable or SUMAVEL Dose Pro?

Individuals who have migraine attacks that:

- Are associated with significant nausea or vomiting
- Rapidly escalate (pain rapidly worsening)
- Occur in the morning (often started in the middle of the night and already moderate to severe upon waking up)

Remember Lisa, the young school teacher, who frequently reported waking up with her menstrual migraines and having to call in sick to work? She may benefit from the quicker onset of action of injectable sumatriptan. With this treatment option, she could feel better in 10–15 minutes and go to work.

Many patients appreciate the convenience of an oral medication for most of their migraine attacks but like having a quick-onset option, such as an injection, for their more severe migraine attacks. The goal is to build a toolbox of different medications and delivery systems to match the right treatment to each headache attack.

- *Maxalt (rizatriptan)* is available in a 5 mg and 10 mg tablet. The tablets come in two types: one is a standard tablet that is swallowed with water; the other (Maxalt MLT) rapidly melts on the tongue when taken. It has a mint-like flavor when dissolved. However, it is not "sublingual" (placed under the tongue), and it does not work immediately, like a nitroglycerine tablet that patients might take for chest pain. It does offer the advantage of not needing water to accompany the dose. Maxalt is considered a short-acting triptan. It can be repeated after 2 hours and then again in another 2 hours. The maximum daily dose is 30 mg. Recently, Maxalt received FDA approval for use in the pediatric and adolescent patient for acute migraine attacks.
- *Relpax (eletriptan)* is available in a 40 mg tablet. It can be repeated after 2 hours to a maximum daily dose of 80 mg. It is a short-acting triptan.
- *Zomig (zolmitriptan)* is available in a 2.5 mg and 5 mg tablet. The oral tablet can be repeated after 2 hours; the maximum daily dose is 10 mg. Like Maxalt, it is available in a rapidly dissolving tablet; in this form, it is called Zomig ZMT and is orange-flavored. Like Maxalt MLT, the Zomig ZMT offers the advantage of not needing water to take but does not offer quicker onset of action than the oral tablet that is swallowed with water. Zomig also comes in a 5 mg nasal spray. The nasal spray, similar to the Imitrex nasal spray, offers quicker onset of action than oral tablets and can be useful for those migraine attacks associated with nausea, vomiting, and/or rapidly escalating pain. The most common side effect of the nasal sprays is a bad taste in the mouth, which for most is worth putting up with if the headache is banished. The onset of action for the triptan nasal sprays (both Imitrex and Zomig) is 15 minutes. However, they are not considered as effective as the injectable sumatriptan.

Which Triptan Is Best?

The best triptan is the one that works best for a particular patient and for that specific migraine attack. For example, I have patients who prefer Imitrex, whereas others feel Relpax works better and others like Frova (frovatriptan). The goal for you is to work with your health-care provider to find the acute migraine treatment that best meets the desired goals of:

- Headache free and back to full function in 2 hours
- No need to redose
- No need to rescue with another medication
- Headache does not come back for at least 24 hours
- The medication is well-tolerated

Triptan-NSAID Combination Tablet

In 2008, Treximet, the first triptan-NSAID tablet was introduced in the United States. Treximet consists of 85 mg sumatriptan with 500 mg naproxen sodium. Since each individual component has been found effective for the acute treatment of migraine, putting them together makes sense. But to be FDA approved, studies had to document that this combination tablet was superior to the individual medications given alone, and that the medication was safe and well-tolerated. The studies were successful, and Treximet was FDA approved. Specifically, researchers found that sumatriptan is rapidly absorbed and is most likely helpful in quickly taking the headache away (often in 1 hour), whereas the naproxen sodium is released slowly and may help prevent the headache from coming back.[8]

Treximet is taken as a single tablet and may be repeated after 2 hours to a maximum of two tablets in 24 hours. It can be taken with or without food. In my experience, it has been a very good medication for migraine attacks and represents an advantage over taking a triptan alone.

Should you consider a change to Treximet or one of the triptans? Ask yourself the following: With my current acute treatment for my migraine attacks,

- Am I consistently headache free in 2 hours?
- Do I have to repeat the dose?
- Do I have to rescue with another medication, such as Vicodin or Fioricet?
- Does the headache go away and stay away for 24 hours?
- Am I clear-headed, alert, and able to function after taking my acute treatment?

If your acute migraine medication does not achieve those goals, you may want to consider a change.

Ergots and Ergot Alkaloids

The ergots and ergot alkaloid class of migraine medication is considered migraine specific but not as specific as the triptans. Examples of ergot medications include Cafergot (ergotamine-caffeine) and Ergostat (ergotamine).

Ergostat (ergotamine) is a sublingual (dissolves under the tongue) tablet for migraine. It contains ergotamine 2 mg, which can narrow the enlarged and throbbing blood vessels that are part of a migraine attack. Side effects are similar to that of caffeine and can include shakiness, heart racing, elevated blood pressure, and insomnia.

Cafergot (ergotamine-caffeine) is a tablet containing 1 mg ergotamine and 100 mg caffeine. The dosage is two tablets taken at the onset of the migraine attack, and then one tablet repeated every 30 minutes to a maximum of six tablets/per attack and a maximum of 10 tablets per week. It also comes as a rectal suppository containing 2 mg ergotamine with 100 mg caffeine. It is inserted rectally as one suppository, which may be repeated after 1 hour with a maximum of two suppositories per attack and a maximum of five suppositories per week. The suppository form can be useful for migraine attacks associated with nausea and vomiting.

This class of ergot medication for migraine is vasoconstrictive, which means it narrows blood vessels, and it can prolong contractions of the uterus during pregnancy and interfere with blood flow to the placenta (and fetus). This class of medication is not considered safe during pregnancy, so it should only be considered if there is no chance of pregnancy. The triptan class is the preferred migraine-specific medication for most female migraine patients. However, those whose migraines don't respond to triptans might find ergots more effective for migraine attacks.

Dihydroergotamine (DHE) medications include Migranal nasal spray and DHE-45, an injectable and intravenous (IV) medication. DHE does not come in an oral form. Migranal nasal spray delivers 0.5 mg dihydroergotamine per spray and is dosed as one spray in each nostril, repeated in 15 minutes in each nostril, to a total dose of 2 mg. The maximum dose is six sprays in 24 hours and eight sprays per week. DHE-45 is given as an injection or in an IV bag and can be very useful in the emergency room or hospital setting. The usual dose is 0.5–1 mg per dose, and this can be repeated every 8 hours. It is often given to help rescue a severe migraine that has been going on for days. It is also used when patients are admitted, and it can help them get off narcotic medication such as Vicodin, Demerol (meperidine), Dilaudid (hydromorphone), Fiorinal (butalbital-aspirin-caffeine), and Fioricet (butalbital-acetaminophen-caffeine). A common side effect is nausea, so patients are often given an antinausea medication such as Reglan (metoproclamide) or Zofran (ondansetron) before the DHE is given.

Ergot alkaloid medications are primarily prescribed for those whose migraines don't respond to triptans and for rescue when a patient is many days into her migraine. Currently, all ergots and ergot alkaloid medications are "Category X" for pregnancy (see Chapter 8) and should be avoided in women of child-bearing years.

Levadex (dihydroergotamine) is an orally inhaled form of DHE that is being developed by MAP Pharmaceutical. It is in clinical trials and is not yet FDA approved. It offers the quick onset of action (10 minutes) of injectable DHE-45 but without the nausea and without a needle. It could prove to be very useful for those who don't respond to triptans, and when quick onset of action is needed. It may also be very helpful for patients who are days into their migraine and need a nonoral form of rescue. Additionally, it may be useful in helping patients get off narcotics or other medications that are creating rebound headache. Studies show that the dihydroergotamines do not have the same safety concerns as the ergots in pregnancy. Therefore, Levadex may have a more favorable pregnancy category rating than the currently available ergots and ergot alkaloids.

In summary, the triptans and ergot alkaloids, including dihydroergotamine, are considered migraine-specific for the acute treatment of migraine attacks. They should be considered first-line therapy for the acute treatment of moderate to severe migraine attacks. The NSAIDs such as naproxen sodium, ibuprofen, and diclofenac may be considered first-line treatment for mild-moderate migraine attacks. Cambia (diclofenac) is the only NSAID approved for the acute treatment of migraine attacks

> ### Box 5-7
>
> What will it take for the migraine attack to go away and stay away? In general, using a migraine-specific agent like a triptan early in the migraine attack is the best way to be headache free in 2 hours and stay headache free for at least 24 hours.

Nonspecific Prescription Medications Used for Headache

Butalbital

Butalbital-containing medications, such as Fiorinal (butalbital-aspirin-caffeine), Fioricet (butalbital-acetaminophen-caffeine), Esgic (acetaminophen-butalbital-caffeine), and Phrenilin (butalbital-acetaminophen), are available as oral tablets and are commonly prescribed for migraine and tension headache. Some are combined with caffeine and some with codeine. The most commonly prescribed butalbital are Fioricet or Fiorinal. Both contain butalbital and caffeine; the third ingredient in Fioricet is acetaminophen (Tylenol) and the third ingredient in Fiorinal is aspirin. Each is dosed as one or two tablets every 4–6 hours as needed for headache.

Butalbital is a barbiturate and highly addictive. It can also cause sedation (sleepiness) and should not be taken if driving or when alertness is needed on the job. It is one of the most common medications to cause rebound headache. The following story is all too common:

Anna, at the age of 29, was given a prescription for 30 tablets of Fioricet when she complained to her gynecologist about her menstrual headaches. Initially, the 30 tablets lasted for 3–4 months and she only needed 1–2 tablets a day for her menstrual headaches. Then, over the next 2 years, she found she needed more and more to get the same benefit. Soon she was calling for refills every 1–2 months. After 2 years, she was requesting 30 tablets every month. After 3 years she was requesting 30 tablets every 2 weeks. Her headache pattern is now an almost daily low-grade headache in addition to her more severe menstrual headaches. The Fioricet helps, but the headache often comes back in 6 hours. The doctor's office continues to refill her Fioricet prescription.

Ten years later Anna, now 39 years old, is in a bad place. She averages 4–5 Fioricet a day, and needs 120–150 tablets a month. Her life is miserable, but she does not know how to get rid of her headaches. She knows the Fioricet is not working as well as it used to, but every time she tries to cut down or stop it, the headaches are bad. She's now struggling with her work and home life. Her headaches are part of her daily life. Her husband and kids are frustrated that she's often missing out on family activities. Her work is suffering, and her boss has called her in and is concerned about missed work days due to headache and her lack of focus and concentration at work when she has a headache. Anna is miserable and depressed. What went wrong?

The situation began with a nonspecific and highly addictive medication prescribed for Anna. If she had been given a triptan (a migraine-specific medication like Imitrex), then it's likely she would not have found herself in this difficult place 10 years later. Anna now has chronic daily headache complicated by medication (Fioricet) over-use. She initially had episodic menstrual headaches, or menstrual migraine, but she has "transformed" into a much more difficult head-ache-prone individual with associated depression. Patients like Anna make up the majority of those we see in headache clinics across the country.

Narcotics and Opioids

Narcotics and opioids are strong pain medications that include codeine, Vicodin (hydrocodone), OxyContin and Percocet (both oxycodone), morphine, Demerol (meperidine), Darvocet (propoxyphene), Dilaudid (hydromorphone), and Stadol nasal spray (butorphanol). Highly addictive, this class of medication is not FDA approved

> **BOX 5-8**
>
> Butalbital-containing medications are *not* recommended for the acute treatment of migraine, including menstrual migraine. If you take a medication like Fioricet or Fiorinal, talk to your healthcare provider about alternative nonaddictive acute migraine medications like the triptans.

for the acute treatment of migraine. Some headache specialists avoid prescribing any of these pain medications for headache because of the severe addictive and rebound headache problems associated with their use. In addition, using this class of pain medication can make a person's headache much more difficult to treat. It is like tasting a very rich chocolate dessert every day, and then having to switch to sugar-free Jell-O or fresh fruit for dessert instead. The brain gets used to the strong pain medication and would not be as "satisfied" with a milder medication, similar to the less-satisfying feeling of a sugar-free dessert compared to the "real" dessert.

Do I ever prescribe this class of medication to my patients? Is it okay to take these medications for severe menstrual migraine?

My answer is a qualified yes: Only in certain cases, and only in limited amounts. I prefer to do everything I can to prevent the disabling migraine (more about that in the next section on mini-prevention) and to minimize the need for pain medication. However, despite our best efforts at preventing and treating menstrual migraine, there are times when the headache may be so severe that having a home rescue with a narcotic or opioid may be necessary. Here are a few examples:

> *Rachel is a 39-year-old woman with four kids. She is separated from her husband and under a lot of stress. Most of her migraines are treated with a triptan and are gone in 2 hours. However, on occasion, her menstrual migraine is so severe that she is vomiting and afraid she will have to go the emergency room. I have taught her how to self-administer an injection of Dilaudid 1 mg on these rare occasions. She gets a prescription for 10 injections every 6 months.*
>
> *Carla is a 48-year-old woman who is an executive and travels a lot in her work. The time change, disruption in her sleep schedule, and stress of travel are triggers for her migraines. She can treat most of her migraines with Treximet (a triptan-NSAID medication), but on rare occasion she rescues with Stadol nasal spray: one spray, one nostril. She only uses it once every other month and feels this saves her from having to go to the emergency room.*

Are there better ways to rescue when the migraine, including menstrual migraine, is very severe? Yes. These will be addressed in the rescue section of this chapter. However, in some cases, the less addictive rescue treatments are not effective or are not well-tolerated, and so this class of narcotics and opioids may be necessary.

> **Box 5-9**
>
> The narcotic and opioid class of pain medication is best avoided when treating acute migraine. It may be useful in a small group of individuals when nothing else works. But these medications should never be used frequently as they are highly addictive and can lead to rebound headache.

Antiemetics (Antinausea) Medications

Antiemetics can be very useful when treating migraine. Many migraine attacks are associated with nausea and vomiting. In addition, antinausea medications can often help the headache pain and, in some cases, may be a reasonable first-line treatment for migraine. Examples of antiemetics include Compazine (prochlorperazine), Phenergan (promethazine), Reglan (metoclopramide), Thorazine (chlorpromazine), Tigan (trimethobenzamide), Vistaril (hydroxyzine), and Zofran (ondansetron). These medications come in a variety of forms including oral tablets, disintegrating tablets, oral solutions, rectal suppositories, and injections. They are commonly given as an injection form or by the IV route when migraines are treated in an urgent care center, emergency room, or hospital setting.

Zofran (ondansetron) and Reglan (metoclopramide) both have Category B ratings for pregnancy, making this class of medications very useful for women who are pregnant or trying to get pregnant. (See Chapter 8 for more specific information on treating migraine during pregnancy and for a complete explanation of the pregnancy category rating system.)

Many of the migraine-specific medications like the triptans help alleviate the nausea that comes as part of the migraine attack. As a result, not as many of my patients need antinausea medication for their acute migraine attacks. However, for some, it is very useful to have an antinausea medication as part of their "migraine toolbox."

Other Nonspecific Acute Migraine Medications

Nonspecific medications to treat acute migraine include Midrin (iso metheptene-dichlorphenazone-acetaminophen), prednisone (a steroid), and Benadryl (diphenhydramine).

Midrin, a combination capsule, contains three medications in each capsule: a vasoconstrictor (which narrows blood vessels) called isometheptene, a sedative (dichlorphenazone), and acetaminophen (Tylenol). It is FDA approved to treat tension and migraine headaches. When treating tension headache, the usual dose is one or two capsules every 4 hours to a maximum of eight capsules in a day. When treating migraine headaches, the usual dose is two capsules initially, and then one capsule every hour to a maximum of five capsules in 12 hours. Midrin is not considered migraine-specific and, in general, is not as effective in treating acute migraine attacks as the triptans. Drowsiness is a frequent side effect due to the sedative component dichlorphenazone.

Over the years, many of my headache patients have taken Midrin. Prior to 1993, when Imitrex (sumatriptan) was introduced, Midrin was considered a reasonable choice for acute treatment of migraine, including menstrual migraine. However, when given a triptan like Imitrex, most of my migraine patients stopped taking Midrin. Many felt that, with Imitrex, they were more clear-headed than with Midrin, which made them drowsy. It is doubtful that Midrin will be the best choice to meet your treatment goals.

Prednisone is a steroid and, with its anti-inflammatory properties, can be very useful in "breaking" a prolonged attack of migraine, including menstrual migraine. It is common to use a course of steroids in oral, injectable, or IV forms for a severe allergic reaction or an asthma attack, but steroids do have side effects, including stomach irritation and skin bruising. Prednisone can also cause bloating (fluid retention) and weight gain, so it should only be used when necessary and for a brief period. It is given in a tapered dose, with a larger amount being taken the first few days to get the headache under control and then the dosage is slowly decreased. It does not cause drowsiness, so it can be an option for women who need to stay alert while taking a migraine treatment. In fact, steroids can cause insomnia, so they are best taken during the day and not at night. Prednisone is generic and reasonably priced. A common course of treatment that I may prescribe is:

- Prednisone 60 mg a day for 3 days
- Prednisone 40 mg a day for 3 days
- Prednisone 20 mg a day for 3 days
- Prednisone 10 mg a day for 3 days

A shorter 3-day course of a steroid called Decadron is often dosed as:

- Decadron 12 mg on Day 1
- Decadron 8 mg on Day 2
- Decadron 4 mg on Day 3

Benadryl (diphenhydramine) is an antihistamine that is available both over-the-counter and as a prescription. It comes in oral form as well as an injectable. It can be used for acute migraine attack, usually in addition to other more specific migraine treatment. It can cause drowsiness, which can be useful if sleep is desired to help treat a severe migraine attack. The normal adult dose is 25–50 mg orally or a 25 mg injection or as an IV treatment given in the emergency room.

Acute Migraine Treatment: A Summary

- NSAIDs, such as ibuprofen, naproxen sodium, and Cambia (diclofenac) may be an appropriate treatment of mild-moderate migraine attacks. Aspirin and acetaminophen may be helpful for a small number of migraine attacks.

- Triptans are the preferred medications for moderate to severe migraine attacks. Dual therapy, such as combining a triptan with an NSAID, may be more effective in some patients than single therapy with a triptan by itself.
- Dihydroergotamine may be useful in triptan nonresponders and to treat medication overuse or rebound headache.
- Butalbital-containing products are best avoided for the treatment of migraine attacks because of their high addictive potential and the problem of rebound headache.
- Excedrin (acetaminophen-aspirin-caffeine) should be limited to a maximum of 2 days a week to prevent rebound.
- All acute medication, including the triptans, should ideally be limited to a maximum of 2 days a week. Even the triptans have been associated with rebound headache.
- Narcotics and opioids should only be used in extreme situations, such as severe migraine attacks not responding to less-addictive medications.
- Prednisone and Toradol (ketorolac) can be helpful when the migraine attack is not responding to initial treatments such as the triptans. Toradol can be administered as an injection or intravenously when migraine is severe.

Short-Term Prevention

Here, we discuss the mini-prevention (or short-term prevention) treatment of migraine headaches, with the focus on short-term prevention of menstrual migraines. Many migraine attacks come out of nowhere and are impossible to treat until the headache is present. However, with menstrual migraine, there is predictability in most cases and short-term prevention can be very useful in preventing or reducing the severity and duration of the menstrual migraine attack.

Short-term prevention refers to preventive treatment that is taken for a limited number of days to prevent migraine attacks. It is ideal for menstrual migraine. A woman can begin preventive treatment several days before her anticipated menstrual migraine and continue until menstruation is complete. Treatment is targeted to the vulnerable time of her cycle. Many women like this approach. For many, their menstrual migraines are described as their worst migraines; the menstrual migraines often are more severe and last longer than nonmenstrual migraines.

Let's hear Melanie's story:

> *Melanie, 35, has two small children. She has migraine without aura. She suffers from a 3- to 4-day menstrual migraine that usually begins the day before her menstruation. She also gets an occasional migraine at other times of her cycle, when the weather changes or from stress. She is able to take Maxalt (rizatriptan) with good results for her nonmenstrual migraines. However, it does not work as well for her menstrual migraines, and she wonders what else she can take. She is also afraid she will run out of her nine Maxalt tablets a month that her insurance allows. Her cycle is 27–28 days. She had a tubal, so birth control is not needed.*

What options does Melanie have?

Integrated short-term prevention for menstrual migraine often includes:

- An NSAID such as naproxen sodium or ibuprofen
- Magnesium
- A triptan for 3–6 days
- Add-back hormonal therapy in some cases

For many women, a combination of these treatments will get the best results.

Short-Term Prevention with NSAIDs

A study examining treatment with Anaprox DS (naproxen sodium) 550 mg taken twice a day from the seventh day before menstruation to the sixth of menstruation found that the women taking naproxen sodium had significantly lighter headache intensity, shorter duration, and fewer headache days compared to the placebo group.[9] Significantly, 33% of the women in this study were completely headache free.

Other anti-inflammatory agents used as a short-term prevention strategy to prevent menstrual migraine include:

- Ponstel (mefenamic acid) 500 mg twice a day
- Ketoprofen 75 mg three times a day
- Meclofenamate 100 mg three time a day
- Motrin (ibuprofen) 800 mg three times a day

Cambia (diclofenac), an NSAID available in powder form, has recently come to market in the United States and may prove useful for menstrual migraine as either an acute treatment or as short-term prevention. It is delivered in individual packets, called *sachets,* which are mixed with water. It has quicker onset of action than the oral NSAIDs and may work in as little as 15 minutes. Diclofenac has been available in the United States as an oral tablet under the brand name of Voltaren, but the Cambia powder form is new. If the headache is already present, it may be more effective than the oral NSAIDs.

This use of an anti-inflammatory medication can be very helpful in reducing the severity of menstrual migraine but is usually not enough for complete relief. It has the advantage of not being expensive, as most NSAIDs are generic and some are available over-the-counter. The disadvantage is that these medications can cause stomach irritation in some women, although taking medication with food can help. Also, it may not be necessary to start taking NSAIDs a full 7 days before menstruation, as was done in the naproxen sodium study. I instruct my patients to begin 2–3 days before their anticipated menstrual migraine. Taking the NSAID daily during this time of the menstrual cycle can help prevent menstrual cramps as well as migraine headache.

> **Box 5-10**
>
> Consider taking naproxen sodium 220–550 mg twice a day beginning at least 2 days before your anticipated menstrual migraine. Naproxen has a long duration of action and can be taken twice a day. Some of the other NSAIDs may need to be dosed three times a day, making them more inconvenient. Naproxen sodium can be purchased as over-the-counter Aleve 220 mg, and a woman can take two at a time. A better option may be to ask your doctor for a prescription for naproxen sodium 550 mg (Anaprox DS) and take one tablet twice a day. Anaprox is available as a generic so the out-of-pocket cost should be low.

Short-Term Prevention with Magnesium

Magnesium has been shown to be helpful compared with placebo; women have reported fewer days with menstrual migraine and lessened pain. It has also been reported to improve premenstrual syndrome (PMS) complaints.[10]

Magnesium can be taken alone as a supplement or as part of a supplement containing other products. The most common side effect of magnesium is diarrhea, so I usually recommend that my patients start at a lower dose (200 mg a day) and then increase to 200 mg twice a day if they are tolerating the lower dose. Combination migraine preventives that contain magnesium include Migrelief and Migravent. Migrelief contains B_2 (riboflavin) and the herbal feverfew in addition to magnesium. Migravent includes butterbur, coenzyme Q-10, and B_2 (riboflavin) with magnesium. Another combination product is called Trigemin; it contains a long list of ingredients in addition to magnesium.

Box 5-11

Magnesium may prevent menstrual migraine. I recommend 200 mg twice a day, starting mid-cycle or on Day 15 for my female patients who only get migraines around the time of their menses. For women who get migraines outside the menstrual window in addition to their menstrual migraines, I recommend taking daily magnesium as a migraine preventive. Many women may prefer to take a combination supplement that contains other ingredients in addition to magnesium. The only negative side effect is diarrhea in some patients.

Let's revisit Melanie's story. Melanie has severe menstrual migraines that last 3–4 days. They typically start the day before menstruation. She wondered what she can do in addition to taking Maxalt for her migraine attacks. Here is what I recommend:

- Begin naproxen sodium 550 mg twice day, 2 days before her anticipated menstrual migraine and take until the end of her period. Take with food to minimize stomach upset.
- Begin magnesium 200 mg once a day and, if there is no diarrhea after 1 week, increase to 200 mg twice a day. She can either start on Day 15 of her cycle and take until her menses, or she may want to simply take magnesium every day. Most of my patients choose to take it every day. It is available over-the-counter.

Is there anything else we can recommend for Melanie? What about short-term prevention with Maxalt (rizatriptan) or another triptan such as Amerge (naratriptan) or Frova (frovatriptan)? Would this be safe? Would there be any risk of rebound headache from taking a daily triptan for 5–6 days in a row?

Short-Term Prevention with the Triptans

Using triptans to provide short-term migraine prevention has been found to be an effective treatment approach for menstrual migraine. Here's what we know:

Frova (frovatriptan) was studied in a large placebo-controlled trial and was found to prevent menstrual migraine for three cycles in more than 50% of the women who participated.[11] Women who took Frova in the study did not have rebound headaches after the Frova was stopped. For these reasons, and because Frova has a long duration of action compared to the other triptans (26 hours), is a very good treatment approach. In my opinion, it is an ideal medication for the short-term prevention of menstrual migraine.

Is there a drawback to using Frova in this way? Unfortunately, yes: cost. Most insurance companies limit the number of triptan tablets taken per month to nine tablets, and, in the study I've just described, the women used 12 tablets. So, here is what I often recommend in my practice:

1. Take a loading dose of Frova 5 mg on the first day of menstrual migraine
2. Take with naproxen 550 mg or ibuprofen 800 mg if you are not already taking an NSAID in a short-term prevention approach.
3. Take Frova 2.5 mg twice day for the next 3–4 days. Some women may only need the Frova 2.5 mg tablet once a day for menstrual migraine prevention.

By using this approach, women can get by with fewer than 12 tablets for short-term prevention of menstrual migraine. Also, for many women in my practice, I help them get approval from their insurance companies for nine tablets of Frova 2.5 mg a month for their menstrual migraines and another triptan such as Imitrex (sumatriptan) for their nonmenstrual migraines.

It's important to note that Frova is only FDA approved for the acute treatment of migraine with and without aura attacks in adults.

When I prescribe Frova as a preventive, I am going "off-label," but I am comfortable with this as the drug has been well-studied and I feel it is a safe and effective approach.

Amerge (naratriptan) has been studied for short-term prevention of menstrual migraine. In one study, Amerge 1 mg taken twice a day for 5 days was found to be highly effective in preventing menstrual migraine. Women began the Amerge 2 days prior to the anticipated menstrual migraine and took it for a total of 5 days. Fifty percent of the women taking Amerge had no menstrual migraine.[12]

Imitrex (sumatriptan) 25 mg three times a day for 5 days was studied for short-term prevention of menstrual migraine. It was found to be effective, but most women will not be able to get the necessary 15 tablets a month from their insurance companies. An alternative would be 50–100 mg twice a day.

Relpax (eletriptan), 20 mg three times a day for 6 days, was found to be effective in reducing menstrual migraine. In this study, participants began treatment 2 days before the anticipated onset of menses and continued for a total of 6 days. A significant reduction in menstrual migraine activity occurred in 53% of the patients.[13]

Zomig (zolmitriptan), 2.5 mg taken twice a day for 7 days in a study of 217 patients, showed a 55% reduction in menstrual headaches compared to 38% in the placebo group.[14] For 40% of women, no menstrual migraine occurred.

BOX 5-12

Consider the use of a triptan taken daily during the menstrual migraine time of your cycle. If your menstrual migraines begin before your period, then track your cycles on a calendar and ideally begin the short-term prevention with the triptan before your headache begins. For those who do not get their menstrual migraines until their period begins, it may be easier to simply start treatment at the first sign of blood flow.

The main downside of taking a triptan for 5–7 days as short-term prevention for menstrual migraine is the cost and the fact that many insurance companies limit how many triptan tablets women can get each month. Ask your healthcare provider for a long-acting triptan like Frova (frovatriptan) 2.5 mg for you menstrual migraines and for a short-acting triptan like Imitrex (sumatriptan) 100 mg for your non-menstrual migraines. By using this approach, many of my patients have been able to get nine tablets of each triptan per month.

Short-Term Prevention with Hormones

Hormones provide an additional treatment strategy that can be useful in reducing the severity and duration of painful menstrual migraine headache attacks. Studies have shown that the drop in estrogen (estradiol) just before menstruation is a big trigger for menstrual migraine. Estrogen itself is not the enemy in menstrual migraine; rather, it is the drop or change in estrogen levels that triggers menstrual migraine.

By preventing or reducing this drop in estrogen that occurs at the end of the cycle and before menstruation, we can dramatically reduce menstrual migraine in many women.

For women like Melanie who have had a tubal ligation (or if their husband has had a vasectomy), we can offer "add-back estrogen." An effective way to do this is by wearing an estradiol patch or by applying an estradiol gel. I usually have women like Melanie use a Vivelle (estradiol) 0.1 mg "dot" estradiol patch for 2 days before their anticipated menstrual migraine or 2 days before menstruation. The Vivelle dot is very small (hence the name "dot") and can be worn on the lower abdomen or buttocks. The estrogen goes through the skin into the bloodstream and can provide a very even level of estrogen to protect against menstrual migraine. The patch can be taken off after 3–4 days and a new one put on. Usually, two patches are enough when being used in the short-term prevention of menstrual migraine.

In a study examining the effectiveness of this approach, improvement in menstrual migraine was seen using the 100 micrograms (mcg; 0.1 mg) estradiol patch from 4 days prior to menstruation to 4 days after for two cycles.[15] The lower patch strengths were not found to be effective. Estradiol 0.1 mg patches are currently available as the Vivelle 0.1 mg dot and Climara 0.1 mg. The Vivelle dot is changed twice a week, and the Climara patch is changed once a week. Remember that these estrogen patches do not protect against pregnancy. Bleeding will still occur. and there will still be a drop in blood progesterone levels.

In one study, applying an estradiol gel (1.5 mg estradiol) from 2 days before menstruation and continuing for 7 days reduced the duration and severity of menstrual migraines compared with the placebo gel.[16] The gel is typically applied to the inner forearms and dosed daily. In another study using estradiol gel 1.5 mg for short-term prevention of menstrual migraine, there was improvement in menstrual migraine but the migraines returned when the gel was stopped after the second day of menstruation.[17] Therefore, when add-back estrogen is used for short-term prevention of menstrual migraine, it may be important to look at timing and not stop it too soon.

How effective is add-back estrogen?

The results can vary from woman to woman. About 50% of women with menstrual migraine in my practice report benefit using add-back estrogen, such as with the Vivelle patch. I recommend my patients try it for 2 months to see if it helps. If there is no benefit after 2 months, I try other treatment approaches.

Putting It All Together

Melanie was prescribed the following:

- Naproxen sodium 550 mg with instructions to begin with one tablet twice a day for short-term prevention of her menstrual migraine. She will track her menstruation on a calendar and begin the naproxen 2 days before her anticipated menses.
- Frova (frovatriptan) 2.5 mg to take at the first sign of menstrual headache pain. She will take Frova 2.5 mg (or 5 mg as

a loading dose) on Day 1 of treatment and then will take Frova 2.5 mg twice a day for 3–4 more days.

- Magnesium 200 mg twice a day. She can take it all month long for migraine prevention.

Melanie returned for her follow-up visit after 2 months and reported some improvement in her menstrual migraines. But was there anything else she could do to further prevent her menstrual migraines?

She was given samples of Vivelle 0.1 mg estradiol patches and instructed to put on a patch several days before her anticipated menses. She was to change the patch after 3 days, with a total of two patches be used per cycle. She was to then return for a follow-up.

Two months later, she reported her menstrual migraines are more manageable.

Does everyone respond like Melanie did? No. Every woman needs to be evaluated and treated individually. However, I know many women like Melanie in my practice, and many of the readers of this book will benefit from short-term prevention treatment for menstrual migraine.

The four key pieces of this short-term treatment approach are:

- NSAIDs such as Aleve (naproxen sodium) or Motrin (ibuprofen)
- Magnesium
- Triptan taken for 3–7 days
- Add-back estrogen for 3–7 days

A combination of these treatments will be necessary in most women to make a difference in their monthly menstrual headaches.

Are there other short-term prevention treatments? Ergotamine 1 mg twice a day taken for a total of 5 days showed some benefit, as did dihydroergotamine (DHE) nasal spray every 8 hours for 6 days in the treatment of menstrual migraine. However, this treatment approach is limited by concerns about safety during pregnancy with this class of medication. Most headache specialists avoid the ergot class of medication in women of child-bearing years.

Herbal preventives other than magnesium may be useful in the prevention of menstrual migraine. These may include vitamin B_2 (riboflavin) and butterbur. However, other than magnesium, most of these other supplements have not been studied in a short-term prevention strategy. They will be discussed in more detail in the nonpharmacologic treatment chapter.

Daily Preventive Medication

Despite our best efforts with acute and short-term preventive treatment for menstrual migraine, some women are so disabled by their menstrual migraines that a daily preventive medication all month long becomes necessary. Goals of daily preventive treatment include:

- Reduction in headache frequency and severity by at least 50% in 8–12 weeks
- The preventive medication is well-tolerated.
- Better response to acute medication
- Better quality of life, including less worry about migraine in between attacks

Let's hear Christy's story. I first met Christy 2 years ago, when she was referred to me by the local emergency room.

Christy came into my office on a Tuesday afternoon for a headache evaluation. A week earlier, she was outside watching her 16-year-old son, Brian, play baseball. She was sitting in the bleachers with the sun shining onto her face. She felt faint, got up to go the bathroom, and was hit with a pounding headache and nausea. She almost blacked out. Concerned, a friend took her to the local emergency room. A brain scan was done, and she was reassured that the results were normal. She was treated with pain medication and sent home with a prescription for Fioricet (butalbital-acetaminophen-caffeine), with instructions to take one table every 4–6 hours. Several days later, she had a return of

> *the severe headache, went back to the emergency room, and was given more pain medications. Several days later, she began her menstrual period.*
>
> *The emergency room did not give her a diagnosis for her headaches. They simply reassured her that the brain scan was normal, and she did not have a brain tumor. She was afraid her headaches would return.*

After careful evaluation, I diagnosed Christy with menstrual migraine. I began her on a daily preventive medication, Topamax (topiramate), since I did not want her to ever have to visit the emergency room twice in one week again. Topamax is an oral medication FDA approved for migraine prevention. I felt it was important to get migraine prevention on board right away for Christy and not wait for short-term prevention for her next cycle. I was also concerned about the Fioricet (butalbital-acetaminophen-caffeine) prescribed in the emergency room as it is highly addictive and often leads to rebound headache. By putting her on Topamax, it would be easier to get her off the Fioricet.

Daily oral preventive medication can also be useful for women who have nonmenstrual migraines in addition to their menstrual migraine. The purpose of a daily preventive is to reduce both the severity and frequency of migraine headaches. To be considered an effective preventive medication, the frequency and severity of migraine headaches should be reduced by at least 50%, and the benefit should be seen within 8–12 weeks.

What are commonly used daily preventive medications?

The three categories of preventive medication most commonly used for migraine prevention are:

- Antiepileptics
- Antihypertensives
- Antidepressants

Antiepileptic (Antiseizure) Medications

Antiepileptics are commonly used for migraine prevention. Two of them are FDA approved for migraine prevention: Topamax (topiramate) and Depakote (divalproic acid). The typical dose of Topamax for migraine prevention is 50–200 mg a day. Common side effects include a tingling sensation in the hands and feet, some sleepiness (best taken at night), and appetite suppression, which may cause weight loss in some individuals. In addition, it can cause some people to have trouble remembering words the next day, and some may even feel "dopey" or not as mentally sharp as usual (Topamax has been referred to as "dopamax" by some). In my opinion, Topamax is highly effective for migraine prevention and continues to be the most common migraine preventive medication I use in my headache practice. I have never found a more effective daily oral migraine preventive than Topamax.

Depakote (divalproex sodium) is another antiseizure-class medication FDA approved for migraine prevention. The typical dose for migraine prevention is 250–1,000 mg a day. Common side effects include tremor (shakiness), weight gain, nausea, and hair loss. In pregnant women, it can increase the risk for neural tube defects in their babies, so Depakote should not be used if there is any chance of pregnancy. Despite its side effects, Depakote can be extremely effective for migraine headache prevention. It is also often used for chronic daily headache and rebound headache. In addition, it is used for bipolar disorder, so if a migraine patient also has bipolar disorder, Depakote would be a good choice for daily prevention.

Other less commonly used antiepileptic medications for daily migraine prevention include:

- *Zonegran* (zonisamide): 50–400 mg a day. It is sometimes referred to as "Topamax light" as it is less likely to cause the mental slowing often associated with Topamax (topiramate). It can be very effective in some individuals needing daily prevention. Side effects include sedation (sleepiness), so it is best taken at night.

- *Lamictal* (lamotrigine): 25–200 mg a day. It is often used for bipolar disorder and may help prevent migraine for some patients. Common side effects include nausea, fatigue, and a serious rash called Stevens-Johnson syndrome.
- *Keppra* (levetiracetam) 250 mg–3 g a day. Side effects include sedation and dizziness. It is rarely used for daily headache prevention but may be useful with the rare patient who has failed other preventives.

Antihypertensives

Antihypertensives refer to medications used to treat high blood pressure. *Beta-blockers* refer to a specific type of blood pressure medication. Two of the drugs in this category have been FDA approved for migraine prevention: Inderal (propanolol) and Blocadren (timolol). Propanolol is dosed from 60 to 240 mg a day for migraine prevention; it comes in a long-acting form called Inderal LA, which is taken once a day. Inderal LA comes in 60, 80, 120, and 160 mg tablets. Blocadren (timolol) is dosed from 10 to 30 mg a day for daily migraine prevention. Both of these beta-blockers can be useful with individuals who have high blood pressure. Other beta-blockers in this class include:

- Atenolol
- Metoprolol
- Labetalol
- Nadolol
- Pindolol

Side effects of beta-blockers include sedation, dizziness, lower pulse rate, and lowering of blood pressure. It may not be a good idea to take beta-blockers if your blood pressure is already on the low side.

Antidepressants

Antidepressants used for migraine prevention fall into three main categories:

- Tricyclic antidepressants (TCAs) like Elavil (amitriptyline) and Pamelor (nortriptyline) have been used for years for migraine prevention. Common doses of both for migraine prevention are 10–75 mg total daily dose, and they are usually taken at night since they can cause sedation (sleepiness). Dry mouth, constipation, and weight gain are other common side effects. These medications are not FDA approved for migraine prevention but can be very effective in some individuals. They are considered the most effective class of medication for chronic tension-type headache. For migraine patients, they can be a good choice for those who also have neck muscle tightness, insomnia, fibromyalgia, or anxiety.
- Selective serotonin reuptake inhibitors (SSRIs) like Prozac (fluoxetine), Zoloft (sertraline), Paxil (paroxetine), Celexa (citalopram), and Lexapro (escitalopram) are often used for migraine prevention but are generally not considered as effective as the TCAs and the serotonin norepinephrine reuptake inhibitor (SNRI) antidepressants. In fact, the SSRIs can cause headache as a side effect of treatment. This class of antidepressants is often prescribed for PMS, premenstrual dysphoric disorder (PMDD), anxiety, depression, obsessive-compulsive disorder (OCD), panic attacks, and posttraumatic stress disorder (PTSD). See Chapter 4, on common comorbid disorders of migraine, to learn more about these conditions and their treatment in migraine. Common side effects of the SSRIs include sexual dysfunction (decreased libido and difficulty achieving orgasm), fatigue, nausea, weight gain, and apathy.
- Serotonin norepinephrine reuptake inhibitors (SNRIs) include Effexor (venlafaxine), Cymbalta (duloxetine), and Pristiq (desvenlafaxine). This class of antidepressants is considered more effective for migraine prevention than the

SSRIs. Cymbalta is FDA approved for fibromyalgia and did not show any sexual dysfunction or weight gain in women in clinical studies. Side effects of this class of medications include tremor, palpitations, insomnia, and nausea. In general, these medications are best taken in the morning.

Significantly, none of the antidepressants listed is officially FDA approved for migraine prevention. However, they can be very effective for migraine prevention in some patients.

The decision of which daily preventive to use is best made between you and your healthcare provider. Other conditions a woman may have can help in selecting the right daily preventive. For example, if a female migraine patient in my practice suffers from depression, I may pick one of the antidepressants as my choice of a daily migraine preventive. I have had women with migraine, depression, and fibromyalgia; in these cases, I may use a daily medication like Cymbalta (duloxetine) in an attempt to treat three medical conditions with the same medication.

Tolerability of a daily preventive medication can be an issue. Let's look at Lisa, the 25-year-old teacher.

❖

Lisa suffers from menstrual migraines that start 1–2 days before menstruation and can last 3–5 days. She also gets nonmenstrual migraines that can last 24-48 hours with stress and weather change. Lately, her migraines are occurring one to two times a week, and she is frustrated. She takes Imitrex but often runs out of her nine tablets a month covered by insurance.

Lisa was offered a daily preventive, Topamax (topiramate), owing to the frequency of her migraines. Initially, she did well, showing a marked improvement in her migraines. However, she felt tired during the day. She was switched to Zonegran (zonisamide), which worked well without the side effects of the Topamax. She continues to take

Zonegran 200 mg a day with excellent results. Herbal prevention with magnesium and attention to lifestyle is also part of her preventive management program. Her birth control pill, Loestrin 1/30, was continued but changed to a continuous (no placebo) regimen. Her frustration with her migraines has lessened, and she feels she is getting her life back.

Other daily preventive medications include:

- Other antihypertensive classes of medications, such as calcium-channel blockers (for example, verapamil), angiotensin-converting enzyme (ACE) inhibitors (for example, lisinopril), and angiotensin receptor blocker (ARB) medications (for example, Atacand/Candesartan). None of these is FDA approved for migraine prevention, but any one may be useful for some individuals who cannot tolerate the beta-blockers, antidepressants, or antiepileptic migraine preventive medications previously discussed.
- Birth control treatments, such as the birth control pill, which can even out the ups and downs in estrogen and progesterone levels that can trigger menstrual migraine. This treatment will be discussed in detail in Chapter 6, on estrogen. This treatment is especially important for women wanting or needing contraception.
- Atypical antipsychotics such as Zyprexa (olanzapine) have been reported to show success in migraine prevention.
- Muscle relaxants such as Flexeril (cyclobenzaprine) and Zanaflex (tizanidine) can be helpful for daily migraine prevention, especially for those suffering from headaches more than 15 days a month. Tizanidine has been shown to be effective in studies of chronic daily headache. It is typically dosed from 2 to 36 mg a day, and it is best given at night due to its sedative side effect.
- Herbal preventives for migraine include magnesium, B_2 (riboflavin), coenzyme Q-10, butterbur, and feverfew.

These will be discussed in more detail in Chapter 7, on nonpharmacologic treatment

Botox for Migraine Prevention

Botox (botulinum toxin) injections for migraine individuals suffering from headache 15 or days a month was FDA approved in October 2010. This can be an option for women who are having frequent headaches despite oral preventive treatment or who have intolerance to multiple preventive medications. Botox can take 2 weeks to be effective and, once effective, lasts for 3 months in the majority of migraine patients. However, not everyone responds to Botox. Until it was FDA approved, the majority of insurance companies would not cover the use of Botox for migraine prevention, and it was cost-prohibitive for most patients. With this recent FDA approval of Botox for migraine prevention, more women will be able to take advantage of this preventive treatment option. Botox can be very effective, especially if combined with other preventive treatment including nonpharmacologic options. It is best suited for women suffering from headaches outside the menstrual time of the month in addition to menstrual migraines. If women only get migraines with menstruation, they probably would not meet the criteria for Botox approval. In my practice, Botox injection has become a common procedure for patients suffering from headache 15 or more days a month. Most patients tolerate this procedure well.

When All Else Fails . . .

Claire, the dental hygienist who works for Kate, has followed all medical advice for her menstrual migraines. She now uses Treximet (sumatriptan-naproxen sodium) for her migraines and tries to take it early in her migraine, as instructed. She takes magnesium 200 mg twice a day for prevention. However, several times a year, her menstrual migraine is so severe she has to go the emergency room and get a pain medication injection (usually Dilaudid [hydromorphone]) and an antinausea medication like Compazine (prochlorperazine) or Phenergan (promethazine). What other options can she be offered for rescue?

Rescue Options for Severe Menstrual Migraine

- Nonoral treatment, such as Imitrex (sumatriptan) 4–6 mg injectable
- Nonoral treatment with Toradol (ketorolac) 60 mg injectable
- Oral treatment with Cambia (diclofenac) powder dissolved in 1 oz of water
- Nonoral treatment with Migranal (DHE) nasal spray
- Rectal suppository of Compazine 25 mg
- Brief course of steroids (e.g., prednisone)
- Intravenous treatment with magnesium, DHE, antinausea medication (such as Zofran [ondansetron]), Toradol, steroids, and/or Benadryl (diphenhydramine); this can often be done in an outpatient setting such as a headache center or an IV infusion center, or in the emergency room.

Claire came to see me and I instructed her on the use of the needle-free Imitrex 6 mg injection for acute treatment of menstrual migraine. She had good results and has not had to visit an emergency room in over 2 years. She continues to use the oral Treximet if her migraine is moderate, but when severe or if associated with nausea or vomiting, she self-injects with the Sumavel Dose Pro 6 mg and is headache free in 15 minutes. She is happy—as is the dental office where she works. No longer does the office have to reschedule patients because of her disabling menstrual migraines. Her insurance allows her to get nine Treximet tablets a month and six Sumavel Dose Pro injections. She feels she has her life back.

Conclusion

For most women, a combination of acute and short-term prevention treatment of menstrual migraine can be very successful in lessening the impact of menstrual migraine. Attention to lifestyle, including good health habits, also should be part of the treatment. Monitoring progress by keeping a headache diary or calendar can also be very helpful.

Daily preventive treatment may be needed for women having frequent and/or disabling migraines. The dose of the daily preventive may, in some cases, need to be increased around the time of menstruation for optimal prevention of menstrual migraine. For example, a woman might take a 50 mg dose of Topamax (topiramate) every night for daily migraine prevention, but increase to 100 mg several days before her anticipated menstrual migraine and continue the higher dose until the end of her period.

As this chapter is brought to a close, I encourage you to evaluate your current treatment plan for your menstrual migraines.

Box 5-13

- Are you headache free and back to full function in 2 hours after your acute treatment?
- Do you stay headache free for at least 24 hours after acute treatment?
- Are you trying short-term prevention with magnesium, an NSAID such as naproxen sodium, a triptan, or add-back estrogen?
- Do you need or want contraception to help your menstrual migraines? (If so, see Chapter 6 on estrogen to learn more about this treatment approach.)

My goal is to eliminate the suffering and disability that menstrual migraine brings into your life. While there is no cure for migraine, there are many very effective treatment approaches that can make a big difference in helping you live a life as headache free as possible. I hope this treatment chapter will help you work with your healthcare provider in developing a treatment plan that, despite menstrual migraine, gives you the freedom to live your life.

References

1. Prior MJ, Codispoti JR, Fu M. A randomized, placebo-controlled trial of acetaminophen for treatment of migraine headache. Headache. 2010; 50: 819–833.
2. Lipton RB, Stewart WF, Ryan RE, et al. Efficacy and safety of acetaminophen, aspirin, and caffeine in alleviating migraine headache pain: three double-blind, randomized, placebo-controlled trials. Arch Neurol. 1998; 55: 210.
3. Diener HC, Bussone G, de Liano H, et al. Placebo-controlled comparison of effervescent acetylsalicylic acid, sumatriptan and ibuprofen in the treatment of migraine attacks. Cephalalgia. 2004; 24: 947–954.
4. Pfaffenrath V, Hans-Christoph D, Pageler L, et al. OTC analgesics in headache treatment: open-label phase vs. randomized double-blind phase of a large clinical trial. Headache. 2009; 49: 638–645.
5. Suthisisang C, Poolsup N, Suksomboon N, et al. Meta-analysis of the efficacy and safety of naproxen sodium in the acute treatment of migraine. Headache. 2010; 50: 808–818.
6. Berenson F, Vasconcellos E, Pakalnis A, et al. Long-term, open-label safety study of oral almotriptan 12.5 mg for the acute treatment of migraine in adolescents. Headache. 2010; 50: 795–807.
7. Brandes J, Cady R, Freitag F, et al. Needle-free subcutaneous sumatriptan (Sumavel Dose Pro): bioequivalence and ease of use. Headache. 2009; 49: 1435–1444.

8. Haberer L, Walls C, Lener S, et al. Distinct pharmacokinetic profile and safety of a fixed-dose tablet of sumatriptan and naproxen sodium for the acute treatment of migraine. Headache. 2010; 50: 357–373.

9. Sances G, Martignoni E, Fioroni L, et al. Naproxen sodium in menstrual migraine prophylaxis: a double-blind placebo controlled study. Headache. 1990; 30: 705–709.

10. Facchinetti F, Sances G, Borella P, et al. Magnesium prophylaxis of menstrual migraine: effects on intracellular magnesium. Headache. 1991; 31: 298–301.

11. Silberstein SD, Elkind AH, Schreiber C, et al. A randomized trial of frovatriptan for the intermittent prevention of menstrual migraine. Neurology. 2004; 63: 261–269.

12. Newman L, Mannix LK, Landy S, et al. Naratriptan as short-term prophylaxis of menstrual associated migraine: a randomized, double-blind, placebo-controlled study. Headache. 2001; 41: 248–256.

13. Marcus D, Bernstein C, Sullivan E, et al. Perimenstrual eletriptan prevents menstrual migraine: an open-label study. Headache. 2010; 50: 551–562.

14. Tuchman MM, Hee A, Emeribe U, et al. Oral zolmitriptan in the short-term prevention of menstrual migraine. A randomized, placebo-controlled study. CNS Drugs. 2008; 22: 877–886.

15. Pradalier A, Vincent D, Beaulieu P, et al. Correlation between oestradiol plasma level and therapeutic effect on menstrual migraine. In: Rose FC, ed. *New Advances in Headache Research*, 4th ed. London: Smith-Gordon; 1994: 129–132.

16. De Lignieres B, Vincens M, Mauvais-Jarvis P, et al. Prevention of menstrual migraine by percutaneous estradiol. Br Med J. 1986; 293: 1540.

17. MacGregor EA, Frith A, Ellis J, et al. Prevention of menstrual attacks of migraine: a double-blind placebo-controlled cross-over study. Neurology. 2006; 67: 2159–2163.

6

Estrogen and Migraine: What Do We Know?

"Estrogen . . . Can't Live with It; Can't Live without It"

Estrogen: curse or blessing? help or hurt for migraine? Good or bad? Just as women are complex in our make-up, the subject of estrogen is complex. Perhaps nowhere in medicine is estrogen more controversial than in the role it plays in the female migraine patient.

Estrogen is a hormone that naturally occurs in women. The primary source of estrogen is a woman's ovaries. When girls are born, they are born with two ovaries, one on each side of the lower abdomen. At puberty, when teenage girls begin having menses, theses ovaries become very active and produce estrogen in a fairly predictable cycle. The ups and downs of estrogen levels are related to migraine occurrence in about 60% of women who have migraines. This 60% figure translates into approximately 12–13 million women migraine sufferers who have a pattern of migraine often being triggered by a particular time in their menstrual cycles.

What is the connection between a woman's own estrogen and migraine? Studies show that the drop in estrogen that occurs during the second half of a woman's cycle (less than 14 days before menstruation) can be a strong trigger for migraine. When the migraine occurs within the 2- to 3-day window prior to menstruation, it is referred to as *menstrual migraine*.

One of the earliest studies establishing the relationship between estrogen and progesterone with migraine was conducted by Dr. Brian Somerville in the early 1970s. It continues to be quoted today. Dr. Somerville studied a group of women migraine sufferers who had a menstrual association with their headaches. He wanted to see what would happen to their migraines if he gave them estrogen versus progesterone late in their cycle, just before menses (see Figure 6-1). Here is what he found:

- When these women were treated with estrogen, the onset of their menstrual migraines was delayed until the estrogen level dropped. They were treated with injectable estradiol.

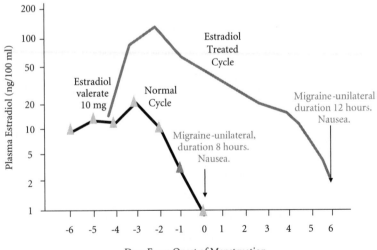

FIGURE 6-1 Estradiol-Treated Cycle. Adapted with permission from Sommerville BW. *Neurology.* 1972; 22: 355–365.

- When these women were treated with progesterone, their bleeding was delayed but not their migraines. In other words, the progesterone did not delay the onset of their menstrual migraines.

Somerville therefore concluded that it is the drop in estrogen that triggers menstrual migraine, as opposed to the drop in progesterone.[1]

Other studies have examined the potential benefit of add-back estrogen in women with menstrual migraine. Add-back estrogen has included estradiol (estrogen) patches, oral estrogen, and topical estrogen. Additional estrogen regimens have included taking hormonal birth control continuously, such as with continuous birth control pills or the contraceptive ring.

Before we describe specific treatments with estrogen used to help migraines, let's step back and look at what estrogen is. To start, estrogen can be divided into *endogenous* estrogen and *exogenous* estrogen.

Endogenous estrogen refers to a woman's own estrogen that is produced from her ovaries. Such estrogens include estradiol, estrone, and estriol. Once a girl reaches puberty, these endogenous estrogens rise and fall in a fairly predictable fashion. When a woman reaches perimenopause (mid-late 40s), levels of hormones fluctuate widely. At menopause (average age 51–52), the ovaries become quiet and no longer produce estrogen, progesterone, and testosterone. Significantly, for many women, migraines go away or improve greatly with menopause.

Exogenous estrogen refers to estrogen that is given to a woman and is not produced by her own body. Exogenous estrogen can be bioidentical (same chemical structure) to what a woman's own ovaries produce or it can be synthetic. The type of estrogen given, the way it is taken, and the dose are highly variable. Exogenous estrogen can dramatically help menstrual migraine, but it can also worsen menstrual migraine. Commonly used preparations are discussed in detail in this chapter.

Let's hear Beth's story.

> *Beth is a 19-year-old woman who has migraine headaches without aura. She typically gets a migraine starting 1–2 days before menstruation that may last for 3–5 days. In addition, she needs birth control. She saw her gynecologist, had a pelvic exam and Pap smear, and was put on a low-dose oral contraceptive pill that had 21 days (3 weeks) of active birth control pill and 7 days (1 week) of placebo. She was instructed to take 1 pill every day and to expect a withdrawal bleed (menstruation) the week of the placebo. Several months later, she noticed an increase in her migraine headaches during her period. She called her gynecologist's office and was advised to stop the birth control pill as it was making her migraines worse.*

Was the birth control pill to blame for Beth's worsening menstrual migraines? Was taking her off it the best advice? Was else could have been done?

Then there is Christy.

> *Christy has suffered with menstrual migraines ever since she was 15. She was put on a successful treatment regimen for years that included the use of naproxen sodium 550 mg twice a day beginning several days before her anticipated menstrual migraine and the use of a triptan for acute migraine. However, now her periods are irregular, and it is harder for her to predict when to start the naproxen. Also, she is getting more headaches at other times of the month, and she is frustrated.*

What is causing Christy's worsening headache pattern? What other questions would we like to ask her?

Last, we have Kate:

> *Kate, who is menopausal, is troubled with hot flashes, night sweats, and insomnia. She also gets migraines. Her migraines were associated with menstruation when she was still having periods, but they stopped at the age of 54. She is afraid to go on estrogen because of all the controversy with breast cancer risk, heart disease, and stroke, but she is miserable with her menopausal symptoms.*

Would putting Kate on estrogen to help her hot flashes, night sweats, and insomnia make her migraines worse or better? Are some types of hormonal estrogen therapy better than others for Kate?

Many patients like Beth want to be on birth control pills. There are many reasons for the use of birth control pills including contraception or birth control; acne; menstrual cramps; irregular and/or heavy menstrual periods; mood swings, such as occur with premenstrual syndrome (PMS) and premenstrual dysphoric disorder (PMDD); and others. What will happen to Beth's menstrual migraines if she goes on the birth control pill? I like to invoke the "one-third rule":

- One-third of patients will notice improvement in their menstrual migraines.
- One-third of patients may see no difference.
- One-third of patients may see a worsening of their menstrual migraines.

Every patient is different in her response to a particular birth control pill, so, unfortunately, there is no way to predict exactly what will happen to Beth's migraines if we put her on the pill. Once she starts, it will become very important to have Beth keep track of her migraines with a headache diary or calendar so we can track her body's response.

What types of birth control can we offer Beth? Here are some options:

- Combined hormonal contraceptive pill: Each active birth control pill includes both estrogen and progesterone. Birth control pills can be divided into *monophasic* and *triphasic* preparations. In monophasic pills, the estrogen and progesterone dose are the same in all the active pills in the pack. In triphasic pills, the estrogen and/or progesterone dose can vary in the active pills. The majority of the estrogen in birth control pills is ethinyl estradiol and ranges from 20 micrograms (mcg) to 35 mcg in most currently used preparations. Ethinyl estradiol is a synthetic (man-made) estrogen. The type of progesterone in most oral contraceptive pills is also synthetic.

- Progesterone-only birth control pills
- Progesterone-only injection (Depo-Provera)
- Estrogen-progesterone contraceptive vaginal ring (NuvaRing)
- Estrogen-progesterone transdermal patch (Ortho Evra)
- Progesterone intrauterine device (IUD) (Mirena)
- Copper IUD (ParaGard)
- Condoms, spermicide, diaphragm

In my opinion, a monophasic, low-dose, combined estrogen-progesterone birth control pill can be very safe for most patients like Beth and may help reduce her menstrual migraines. You may recall that her gynecologist's office advised her to stop taking the oral birth control pill when she noticed a worsening of her menstrual migraines with menstruation. But here is the problem: Her migraines were not worse because of the estrogen in the active pills; they were worse because of the placebo pills! Estrogen is not the enemy in menstrual migraine; for most women, it is the drop in estrogen that is the culprit. Specifically, when Beth begins her placebo week in the birth control pack, her estrogen level drops dramatically and this is the trigger for her worsening migraines.

The amount of estrogen in birth control pills is "supraphysiologic." In other words, it is greater than the amount of estrogen that would normally be present from a woman's own ovaries. This is necessary because the level has to be high enough to block ovulation and prevent pregnancy. Therefore, the drop in estrogen from the active pill to placebo is much greater than the physiologic or natural drop experienced by a woman who is not on birth control pills. This greater drop in estrogen levels explains why Beth's menstrual migraines were worse when she was put on the birth control pill.

How can we help Beth feel better? Can she stay on the birth control pill?

Yes. She can be instructed to skip the placebo week, and instead take 3 weeks of the active pill and then immediately go into her next pill pack. If she skips the placebo week, her estrogen level remains constant, and this may prevent her menstrual migraine completely. Even if she experiences some migraine attacks, the severity would be expected to be less intense if her estrogen level is steady.

Doesn't Beth need to have a period and be "cleaned out" every month"? What will happen to the blood that builds up in her uterus? Won't she have bloating, breast tenderness, and spotting? Is it safe for her to keep taking the active birth control pill? How often should she cycle off and have a withdrawal bleed or period?

Beth does not need to have a period every month when she is on the birth control pill. For most women, the lining of the uterus does not build up to a significant amount in 1 month. In fact, several birth control pills feature a continuous 12 weeks of active pills followed by either 1 week of placebo or 1 week of "add-back estrogen" (such as Seasonale and Seasonique).

Box 6-1

Here's an analogy that may help explain why most women can easily take continuous birth control pills for 3 or more months in a row before cycling off: If a woman is *not* on birth control pills, the lining of her uterus builds up like shag carpet and needs to be cleaned out monthly. If she *is* on birth control pills, the lining of her uterus is more like that thin "indoor-outdoor" carpet and does not need to be cleaned out. A woman's body will usually tell her when she needs to cycle off and bleed if she is taking continuous birth control. In particular, women tell me they begin experiencing bloating, break-through bleeding, or premenstrual symptoms and then can cycle off for 4 days. I recommend limiting the pill-free days to no more than 4 in a row. Going off for 4 days will allow for withdrawal bleeding without causing the estrogen level to drop for a full 7 days, as is typical with most birth control regimens. The prolonged 7-day drop in estrogen that is part of most birth control packs can cause a prolonged menstrual migraine.

Returning to Beth's situation, these are the specific birth control pills I would consider for her: Yaz, Yasmin, Loestrin 24, Mircette, Ovcon, Seasonale, Seasonique, LoSeasonique, or Lybrel. There are countless birth control pills available on the market, and many are generic. You may not see your birth control pill in this list, but knowledge of how each of these work still may be useful for you. Let's explore them in closer detail.

Yaz is a 24/4 (24 active pills followed by 4 placebo pills) monophasic combined estrogen/progesterone birth control pill. Each active pill contains 20 mcg of ethinyl estradiol (a synthetic estrogen commonly referred to as EE) and a synthetic progesterone, drospirenone. It is currently one of the most widely prescribed oral birth control pills in the United States. Women can take all 28 days in the pill pack and have a monthly bleed; this is considered *cyclical use*. Alternatively, they may take Yaz continuously and only cycle off every 3–6 months. To do this, they would take the 24 active pills, skip the last 4 placebo pills, and immediately go into the next active pill pack.

Yasmin is a 21/7 (21 active pills followed by 7 placebo pills) monophasic combined estrogen/progesterone birth control pill. Each active pill contains 30 mcg of ethinyl estradiol with drospirenone. It can be taken cyclically or continuously. In general, there is less break-through bleeding on Yasmin than Yaz due to the higher amount of estrogen. Both preparations are, however, considered "low-dose" birth control. There are now generic versions of Yasmin, so the lower cost can be an advantage over Yaz for some women.

Loestrin 24 is similar to Yaz in that there are 24 active pills followed by 4 placebo pills. The estrogen (ethinyl estradiol) is the same as in Yaz and Yasmin; the synthetic progesterone is different. The synthetic progesterone in Loestrin is norethindrone acetate. In my opinion, there is no major advantage to Loestrin over Yaz, but there can be individual differences in how they are tolerated.

Mircette contains 20 mcg of EE with synthetic progesterone in the first 21 days of the pill pack; this is followed with two placebo pills and then 5 days of "add-back" estrogen with 10 mcg EE but no progesterone in the last five pills. In general, bleeding will occur when the progesterone is left out of the pill. In my practice, I often have a woman with menstrual migraine take the first 3 weeks of the active pill in the pill pack and then immediately go to a new pill pack and take the first 3 weeks in the new pill pack. After 6 weeks of the active pill, I then have her take two of the estrogen-only pills for 5 days. In this way, she is maintaining an even 20 mcg EE throughout her cycle. She will bleed during the 5 days of EE-only pills if the lining needs to be shed since there is no progesterone in the "add-back" estrogen-only pills.

Ovcon 35 has 35 mcg of ethinyl estradiol in the first 3 weeks of the pill pack combined with a synthetic progesterone, and it may have an advantage if women experience break-through bleeding on the 20–30 mcg lower-dose EE formulations. It is considered a monophasic cyclical pill but can be converted to continuous use for women with menstrual migraine.

Seasonale, Seasonique, LoSeasonique, and *Lybrel* are all examples of extended-release forms of oral birth control pills. Seasonale features 12 weeks (72 days) of 30 mcg EE with synthetic progesterone followed by 1 week (7 days) of placebo pills. Seasonique has the same 12 weeks of active pills with 30 mcg EE followed by 1 week of "add-back estrogen" pills. The add-back estrogen pills contain 10 mcg of EE so may offer an advantage in reducing menstrual migraine. However, there is still a drop in EE from 30 mcg to 10 mcg. This drop may still be a trigger for menstrual migraine in women taking Seasonique. LoSeasonique offers 12 weeks of 20 mcg EE with synthetic progesterone followed by 1 week of 10 mcg EE. These extended-release forms of birth control can all be good options for women with menstrual migraine. (Many women also like not having a period every month!)

Lybrel contains a daily continuous regimen of EE and synthetic progesterone for 1 full year. Theoretically, this could prevent menstrual migraine completely by preventing any drop in estrogen, as well as preventing menstrual periods. The drawbacks include break-through bleeding, breast tenderness, and bloating. Some women feel better from cycling off and having a period every 2–3 months.

There are many good options for birth control pills. The bottom line for any woman with menstrual migraine is to be aware that a birth control pill could help, hurt, or not affect her migraines. Keeping a headache diary is critical for monitoring the effect of a particular birth control pill on migraine headaches in a woman.

Are there any reasons why a woman should not take any estrogen-containing form of birth control?

Yes. Women who have had a blood clot (sometimes referred to as a deep venous thrombosis or DVT) or a pulmonary embolism (PE) should not take estrogen. Women who have clotting disorders or any condition that would put them at risk for stroke should not take estrogen-containing contraception. Smoking, uncontrolled high blood pressure, high cholesterol, and obesity all increase the risk of stroke when a woman is on birth control pills. Migraine with aura carries an increase risk for stroke; in general, these migraine patients should not take an estrogen-containing form of contraception. Aura, by definition, refers to the reversible neurological signs and symptoms that about 10–15% of migraine patients experience. Usually, aura is visual and may include zigzag lines, flashing lights, and visual distortions. It can also include the loss of vision. Other aura symptoms may include tingling on one side of the body or slurred speech. For a full description of aura, see Chapter 1.

Patients like Beth have other options for birth control, and these options can affect their migraine headaches.

Mini-Pill

The "mini-pill" refers to oral contraceptive products that contain progesterone only and no estrogen. They are sometimes referred to as "progesterone-only pills" or POPs. They work to prevent pregnancy by changing the cervical mucus. They interfere with the egg and sperm's ability to implant or "settle in" on the uterus. The mini-pill may block ovulation but not as consistently as the combined estrogen-progesterone birth control pill. As a result, there is a higher pregnancy rate with progesterone-only pills. However, they may be a good option for those women migraine patients who can't take estrogen for health reasons or those who find that estrogen aggravates their migraine headaches. In the progesterone-only pill, every pill contains active progesterone; there is no placebo. Bleeding can be irregular. Common name brands include Micronor and Nor-QD.

Depo-Provera

Depo-Provera is an injection of synthetic progesterone (medroxyprogesterone acetate) that is administered into a muscle every 3 months for birth control. It contains 150 mg of progesterone. It can be convenient for women who have trouble remembering to take an oral pill every day or for those who can't take estrogen. However, side effects include headache, depression, and weight gain. I don't like using it in my headache practice because of these side effects. One problem is that if a woman has a side effect from the Depo-Provera, she has to wait 3 months for it to get out of her system.

Ortho Evra

Ortho Evra is a contraceptive patch that contains 20 mcg EE with synthetic progesterone. It is designed to be worn on the skin for 3 weeks and then taken off for 1 week. When it first came on the market, I was excited, thinking this could be a great contraceptive option for my migraine patients. I thought that, since the EE was absorbed through the skin, it would produce a nice even estrogen level. However, after Ortho Evra was on the market and being used by large numbers of women with migraine, it became clear that, for many women, it aggravated their migraines. It was discovered that the level of estrogen was higher soon after a new patch was placed on the skin and then the level would decrease as the patch was due to come off. Patch users may be exposed to 60% more estrogen are than women using a 35 mcg EE oral contraceptive; in addition, the level of estradiol can drop to 25% lower than that experienced with oral contraceptives.[2] The uneven levels of estrogen are thought to be the cause of the migraine aggravation in women using Ortho Evra. As a result, I rarely use this method of contraception in my women migraine patients.

Intrauterine Devices

Intrauterine devices for contraception are placed into the cervical part of the uterus by a trained healthcare professional. There is a progesterone IUD called the Mirena IUD, and there is a nonhormonal IUD called ParaGard (containing copper). IUDs can be a good option for women who can't take estrogen but need birth control. In general, they would not be expected to help or hurt migraine headaches. Side effects can include heavy periods, cramping, and some risk of infection.

Implanon (Progesterone Rod)

Implanon is a progesterone rod that is placed under the skin of the inner arm by a trained healthcare provider. It provides birth control through a continuous release of progesterone. It is removed and a new one inserted every 3 years. The potential advantage of this birth control method is that there it contains no estrogen; therefore, for women migraine patients who cannot take estrogen, this could be a good option if birth control is needed.

Condoms, Spermicide, and Diaphragms

Condoms, spermicide, and diaphragms are nonhormonal means of contraception. Although not as effective as birth control pills, they can be useful in some cases of menstrual migraine. For example, if I have a patient who is unsure if her birth control pill is making her migraines worse, I may recommend she switch to condoms and spermicide for a few months and watch her migraine pattern. She may prefer to be fit with a diaphragm that would then be used with a spermicide to increase its effectiveness for birth control.

❖

There are many birth control options for women with migraine, including those with menstrual migraine. The effect of a particular birth control treatment on a woman's migraine headaches is unpredictable; therefore, it is critical to keep a headache diary and watch what happens to the headache pattern whenever birth control is begun.

Do any studies look at what happens to headaches (and migraines) with different birth control options? What do we know?

One of the problems in birth control clinical trials is that women often were simply asked if they had a headache, leaving the headache undiagnosed as a migraine headache. The package inserts of all birth control pills will list headache as a possible side effect. That may be true. However, I feel that many women migraine patients can benefit from birth control pills, if they are taken the right way. In general, the "right" or best way is to maintain an even estrogen level. As far back as 1997, a study was published in *Obstetrics Gynecology*, a leading journal, discussing the potential benefit of extending the duration of active oral contraceptive pills to manage hormone withdrawal symptoms.[3] More recently, another study published by Dr. Patricia Sulak gives us evidence that continuous oral contraceptive use may be better than cyclical use for women with menstrual migraine.[4] In this study, when the pill was taken continuously, there was a dramatic reduction in the cyclical headache pattern. This study was instrumental in supporting what many of us do clinically in prescribing continuous birth control pills.

In another related study, Sulak and her colleagues observed 80 women and compared cyclical versus continuous use of an oral contraceptive pill in terms of headache, pelvic pain, and mood. Significantly, not only did these women have less menstrual migraine, their mood was better and they had less pelvic pain. Sounds like a "win-win"!

Women often ask me these questions:

- "What if I cannot tolerate continuous oral birth control pills due to too much break-through bleeding?
- "What if I want to cycle off and have a period every month?"
- "What should I do about my migraine when I stop to have a period every 3–4 months?

The answer: Add-back estrogen

Add-back estrogen refers to taking estrogen in an oral or topical form (like a gel or patch) when cycling off an active contraceptive product, such as an oral birth control pill, or when taking out the NuvaRing vaginal ring. The concept is to minimize the drop in estrogen that can cause or aggravate menstrual migraine. This can be done in several ways:

- *Wear an estradiol patch*, such as the Vivelle dot or Climara. In a study of 24 patients with menstrual migraine, a reduction in the frequency of menstrual migraine was observed with the 0.1 mg (100 mcg) dose of estradiol. No significant benefit was observed in women treated with a lower dose 0.025 mg (25 mcg) of estradiol.[5] Another study showed no benefit over placebo when the 0.05 mg (50 mcg) dose of estradiol patch was used.[6] Therefore, it is important to use the higher dose of estradiol patch to see benefit for menstrual migraine. In my practice, I commonly use the Vivelle 0.1 mg estradiol patch and instruct women to change after 3 days. Usually two patches per cycle are enough to prevent the drop in estrogen that occurs with menstruation. I write "do not substitute" so women get the name-brand Vivelle dot patch. From my experience, many women have an allergic skin reaction to the larger, generic estrogen patches. Important caution: Do not confuse the add-back estradiol patch with the Ortho Evra contraceptive patch. The estradiol patches are a lower dose of estrogen and are normally used for hormone replacement in menopausal women. Ortho Evra contains synthetic estrogen (ethinyl estradiol) and synthetic progesterone and should not be used for add-back estrogen in menstrual migraine.

- *Apply an estradiol gel.* Gels have been evaluated in several published studies. However, it was found in a recently published study that stopping the estrogen gel too soon may result in an increase in migraine.[7] In my opinion, the estrogen gel should be continued until menstruation is completed.
- *Take an oral estrogen tablet* during the oral contraceptive, patch, or ring-free week. In a published study, 0.9 mg per day of Premarin (conjugated equine estrogen) was given to women during their hormone-free week; the researchers found a 77% reduction in the number of headache days per cycle.[8]

A patient in my practice came in recently for follow-up of her menstrual migraines. She is on continuous birth control pills and cycles off for 4 days every 3 months. During these 4 days, she often suffered with a 4-day menstrual migraine. We gave her some samples of Vivelle dot 0.1 mg at a visit several months ago (Vivelle contains 0.1 mg estradiol). She now puts this patch on when cycling off her birth control pill and has noticed great improvement. She only needs one patch for the 4 days she cycles off. She is very pleased with her results, and she still has a triptan to take when needed; in her case, she likes Treximet (sumatriptan-naproxen combination).

Many providers may give you a few samples of the Vivelle dot or other add-back estrogen treatment to try during your period. How long do you take to decide if it is helping? I recommend trying for at least two cycles. In my practice, I estimate that add-back estrogen helps in at least 50% of the women I give it to.

Christy's migraines are getting out of control, as are her periods, which are irregular and hard to predict. Now 47 years old, she has suffered from menstrual migraines since she was 15. Until 6 months ago, she was doing well taking naproxen beginning several days before her anticipated menstrual migraine; she took naproxen 550 mg twice a day for 7 days as a mini-preventive. She also took Imitrex (sumatriptan)

> *100 mg for acute treatment when she got a migraine; on occasion she self-injected with Imitrex 6 mg when a menstrual migraine was severe. However, she is now having so many headaches that she is running out of her nine Imitrex tablets a month that her insurance allows. She's frustrated. She's also noticing some insomnia and, on occasion, hot flashes. Her periods are anywhere from 2 weeks to 2 months apart. Her migraines have gotten worse because she is going through perimenopause.*

Perimenopause and Migraines

Perimenopause is the time in a woman's life when her ovaries "go crazy." The estrogen and progesterone levels are all over the place as her ovaries are no longer producing the hormone levels on a regular schedule. Typically, the age of perimenopause begins in the 40s, usually between 45 and 50. It can last for 4–10 years but most often lasts from ages 47 to 51. Studies show that this is a time when migraines often worsen dramatically in women. Women who have a history of menstrual migraine or previous migraine exacerbation related to birth control pills, pregnancy, or postpartum are especially vulnerable to migraines getting worse during perimenopause.[9] This would make sense as these are all times of hormonal change in women.

Does checking hormone levels make sense?

In some cases, yes. Checking estradiol levels, for example, can help determine if a woman is in perimenopause or menopause. An estradiol level is often ordered along with a follicle stimulating hormone (FSH) level. FSH is a hormone produced by the hypothalamus gland in the brain. The FSH level influences the ovary to produce estrogen. As a woman moves into menopause from perimenopause, the FSH increases and the estrogen level decreases. Testing through saliva has become popular; however, I prefer to measure hormone blood levels. It is always important to note where you are in your menstrual cycle, including the day of your last menstrual period, when any hormone level is checked. This can help physicians interpret the data properly.

Would estrogen be helpful for Christy? Is it safe? How should she take it?

To answer these questions, we need more information. We should find out if Christy needs birth control. If she has had a tubal ligation or her husband has had a vasectomy, then we may approach her treatment differently. Unfortunately, many women who are perimenopausal mistakenly assume that their chances of pregnancy are very low. Remember, though, that it only takes one egg to be released at ovulation to get pregnant. It is not uncommon for a woman in her late 40s or even early 50s to go to her doctor to be tested for menopause when she notices that she hasn't had her period in 2–3 months. Surprise—she's pregnant! Never assume, based on age or perimenopausal symptoms, that you do not need birth control.

If Christy doesn't need birth control (for instance, if she had a tubal), here are some options for treatment:

- Start taking a daily preventive such as Topamax (topiramate).
- Consider herbal supplements and lifestyle changes.
- Consider estrogen either as hormonal therapy (HT) or with low-dose contraception if she is healthy, has migraines without aura, or has no major risk factors for stroke or heart disease. (Note: If Christy is a smoker, or if she has uncontrolled high blood pressure, she should not take any form of estrogen.)

Finally, I would reassure Christy that there is "light at the end of the tunnel" in that her migraines may go away or get much less intense when she is menopausal. Doctors and patients need to aggressively treat migraine during perimenopause because of the woman's fluctuating hormone levels (which wreak havoc on migraines), and a patient may feel as if she needs to take more medication that she would like. But she should keep in mind that she will not have to take these medications for the rest of her life. Christy's migraines will improve in the future.

Hormonal Therapy: Options

Hormonal therapy can be taken in the form of a tablet, a gel, a patch, a spray, or even a pellet placed just under the skin. My preference is to use estradiol, a form of estrogen that is bioidentical to that produced naturally by a woman's ovaries. Estradiol is most responsible for preventing hot flashes, night sweats, and other menopausal symptoms. Bioidentical means that the hormone is chemically (and structurally) identical to what is produced by our own bodies. As such, bioidentical hormones are expected to cause fewer side effects. The way I see it, we are simply giving back that which our own bodies no longer sufficiently produce. In Christy's case, her own ovaries are still producing some estradiol but not as much or as evenly as she is used to. If Christy is prescribed a low-dose hormone product, she is not shutting down her own ovaries; rather, she is adding to her own body's production of estradiol.

Specific hormonal estradiol treatment options include:

- Vivelle dot patch: 0.025 mg, 0.0375 mg, 0.05 mg, 0.075 mg, 0.1 mg
- Climara patch: 0.025 mg, 0.0375 mg, 0.05 mg, 0.06, 0.075 mg, 0.1 mg
- Alora patch: 0.025 mg, 0.05 mg, 0.075 mg, 0.1 mg
- Estrogel: 1–2 pumps/day
- Elestrin: 1–2 pumps/day
- Divigel: 1 packet/day
- Estrasorb: 2 packets/day
- Evamist: 1–2 sprays/day
- Oral estradiol (Estrace): 0.5 mg, 1 mg, 2 mg
- Estrogen pellet placed under the skin (in-office procedure)

> **BOX 6-2**
>
> I do not recommend synthetic estrogen products such as Premarin (conjugated equine estrogen) and Ogen. They tend to have more side effects including headache; they go through the liver to be metabolized, unlike nonoral formulations that go directly into the blood system through the skin and thereby produce more even estrogen levels. Finally, Premarin received a lot of negative attention in the Women's Health Initiative Study.

Hormonal therapy is expected to help lessen menopausal symptoms such as insomnia, hot flashes, and night sweats. Could HT help migraines, including menstrual migraine?

Unfortunately, we don't know. Each individual woman varies in her response to HT. One of the problems with HT in a perimenopausal woman is that her own ovaries will continue in their unpredictable pattern until she becomes completely menopausal. The HT we give her does not shut down her own ovaries; we are simply adding a "layer" of estradiol. However, the benefit of improved sleep and fewer hot flashes and night sweats can help with her overall quality of life. Estrogen is also known to help with mood.

Should Christy take cyclical or continuous HT?

My preference would be continuous HT. Cyclic HT can aggravate her already fluctuating estrogen levels and could aggravate her migraines.[8]

Should Christy take progesterone?

It depends. If she is still having a period at least every 2–3 months, then probably I would not give her progesterone. If she goes for more than 3 months without a period, then I may give her a 12-day course of natural progesterone like Prometrium to allow for a withdrawal bleed. There is a slight risk of uterine cancer if the lining of the uterus builds up and there is no cleaning out. This is only a risk in women who still have a uterus. If a woman has had a hysterectomy (had her uterus surgically removed), then progesterone is not necessary.

Would a low-dose birth control pill be an option for someone like Christy, even though she does not need birth control?

Yes. More and more women are now being treated with low-dose birth control pills to help ease their transition from perimenopause to menopause. Birth control pills can help regulate the menstrual cycle and allow for more predictable periods; they can lessen cramping associated with menstruation and make periods shorter and lighter. If a woman is at low risk for stroke and heart disease, then most gynecologists and other healthcare providers will allow her to stay on a low-dose birth control pill until her mid-50s.

Would the low-dose birth control pill help Christy's menstrual migraines more than HT with estradiol?

Maybe. Remember that the birth control pill will "shut down" her ovaries' production of estrogen and progesterone, unlike estradiol hormonal therapy. Her levels of estrogen and progesterone will be higher from taking the birth control pill and, therefore, this may help lessen migraine. Also, by regulating and making her periods more predictable, she can expect more success from the current mini-prevention routine she is following using naproxen and acute therapy with Imitrex (sumatriptan).

How will Christy know when she is menopausal if she keeps taking the birth control pill?

Around the age of 55, Christy should stop taking the birth control pill and see what her body does. After several months, she can have an FSH and estradiol blood level test to help determine if she is still in perimenopause or has entered menopause. This can help her treatment team develop the best treatment plan. Occasionally, someone like Christy is given the "progesterone challenge" when off the birth control pill. This involves taking a progesterone pill like Provera (synthetic progesterone) 10 mg a day for 5–7 days to see if withdrawal bleeding occurs several days after completion of the Provera. She could be given micronized natural progesterone in the form of Prometrium instead of Provera. If there is no bleeding, it suggests menopause. If there is bleeding, it would suggest she is still in perimenopause and that her ovaries are still producing some estrogen. Estrogen is responsible for building up the lining of the uterus.

What else can Christy do?

In addition to hormonal therapy, Christy may benefit from a daily preventive medication. The choice would be determined based on other symptoms and medical conditions she may have. For example, if she needed to lose weight and was having trouble sleeping, Topamax (topiramate) would be a good choice, based on its potential side effects of appetite suppression and sedation (sleepiness). If neck tightness or fibromyalgia was present, then tricyclic antidepressants like Elavil (amitriptyline) or Pamelor (nortriptyline) may be better choices. If hot flashes and night sweats are present, then Effexor (venlafaxine) or Cymbalta (duloxetine) may be preferred. (Effexor has been shown to decrease hot flashes in clinical studies).[10] Other medications shown to decrease hot flashes include Prozac (fluoxetine)[11] and Neurontin (gabapentin).[12] Although not FDA approved to prevent migraine, these medications (Cymbalta, Effexor, Prozac, and Neurontin) have shown benefit for migraine in clinical studies. With any preventive, it is important to start at a low dose to watch for side effects. In most cases, the patient can slowly increase the dose to get the maximum benefit.

A patient like Christy should see her doctor more often for follow-up due to exacerbation of migraine during perimenopause.

Menopause and Migraine

Now let's turn our attention to Kate.

Let's return to Kate and her situation. Should Kate go on estrogen? The short answer is that there is no clear-cut answer. A couple of years

Kate is a 55-year-old woman in menopause. She is suffering from typical menopausal symptoms like hot flashes, insomnia, and night sweats. However, she is afraid to go on estrogen because of her history of menstrual migraines, which are finally better now that she is no

longer having periods. She has not had a period for 15 months. She is still getting an occasional migraine headache but is finally free of her disabling menstrual migraines!

Kate's migraines are better. This makes sense since her hormone levels (mainly estrogen and progesterone) are no longer wildly changing. In general, migraines improve during menopause. However, the improvement is seen more in women who go through menopause spontaneously (i.e., on their own). If they are thrown into menopause through surgery (with ovaries being removed), their migraines may worsen. A study of menopausal women showed that two-thirds of women with migraine improved, with less migraine in menopause. However, only one-third improved if their menopause was caused by surgical removal of their ovaries.[13]

Box 6-3

Having your ovaries removed to get rid of menstrual migraines is *not* a good idea. The dramatic drop in estrogen can be aggravating for migraines. It is much better to gradually go through menopause and let your ovaries slowly produce less estrogen. The hot flashes, night sweats, and insomnia are no fun, but we can offer treatment to help these symptoms in a way that won't aggravate migraines.

Box 6-4   Personal Note

What have I chosen for myself during perimenopause and now menopause? Realizing that all of us are unique, and my choice may not be your best choice, here is what I did: I took low-dose continuous birth control pills until the age of 53. I then decided to go off and see what my body wanted to do. After several

(continued)

Box 6-4 (continued)

months of no period but lots of hot flashes and night sweats, I went in for a complete physical and blood work. My FSH level was high and my estradiol level was low, indicating menopause. I then tried different topical estradiol treatments, and I have chosen a gel that I rub on my inner arms once a day. I like that it is bioidentical to what my ovaries used to produce. How am I doing? I am happy to answer that I am currently doing great. I no longer suffer from menstrual migraines. On occasion, I still get a migraine for which I take a triptan (Treximet, a suma-triptan-naproxen combination) as needed. Still, I can now go for weeks without a migraine! My current migraine triggers are no longer hormonal ups and downs; rather, they are stress and lack of sleep. I am trying to control those, although not always successfully.

ago, the Women's Health Initiative created a lot of fear among women in suggesting that estrogen was dangerous.[14] Keep in mind that there were many flaws in this study, including the fact that the average age in the study was 63 and that only synthetic estrogen (Premarin) and synthetic progesterone (Provera) were used. Therefore, the results of this study may not apply to perimenopausal women or to women early in menopause. Also, the results should not be applied to other forms of HT including those using bioidentical estradiol and proges-terone preparations.

The decision of whether to go on estrogen is an individual one, one that needs to take into account individual risk factors such as per-sonal or family history of breast cancer, heart disease, stroke, clotting disorders, and any other conditions for which estrogen would be a problem.

Potential benefits for HT include relief of hot flashes, night sweats, and insomnia (all common menopausal symptoms); treatment or prevention of osteoporosis; and relief of moderate to severe vaginal dryness that is unresponsive to topical treatment. Many health-care providers, as well as leading national organizations such as the American College of Obstetrics and Gynecology and the National Menopause Society, have adopted the following general recommendation: Use the lowest dose of estrogen for the shortest amount of time necessary to treat the symptoms.[15,16]

Will estrogen HT aggravate Kate's migraines?

We're not sure. What we do know is that oral synthetic estrogen (like Premarin) would be more likely to aggravate her migraines than would transdermal estradiol. A published study showed increased migraines with oral estrogen HT compared to transdermal HT.[17] One theory is that the transdermal (patch) delivery gets the estrogen directly into the bloodstream, thus creating a more even estradiol level than the oral estrogen does, which has to go through the liver to be metabolized.

Kate is in early menopause. She is suffering with hot flashes, night sweats, and insomnia. If she had no major risk factors for estrogen, then her treatment options would include:

- Estradiol low-dose in a patch or gel; for example, the Vivelle dot 0.025 mg patch (she would change the patch twice a week).
- Prometrium 200 mg Days 1–12 (first 12 days of every month). Prometrium is natural micronized progesterone and is bioidentical.

Kate should come back to visit her doctor in 2 months. If she were still having hot flashes and night sweats, I would increase the dose of her Vivelle patch. She would be encouraged to keep up with regular Pap smears, mammograms, and bone health (DEXA) tests for osteoporosis screening, and with blood work that should include a vitamin D level. Blood work could also include an estradiol level to help assess the dose of the estradiol patch she is wearing. Some providers like following estradiol levels in menopausal women; others prefer to simply review how a woman is doing in terms of how well her symptoms are being managed with a given dose of estrogen.

What if Kate has a strong family history of breast cancer?
In that case, I may suggest she take phytoestrogens instead of estrogen prescription products. The word "phyto" means plant; phytoestrogens are plant-derived substances that have estrogen-like activity and may help with hot flashes, night sweats, and insomnia. Black cohosh, red clover, and soy are examples of phytoestrogens. In addition, Kate could be offered a medication like Effexor (venlafaxine). For her insomnia, a sleeping medication like Ambien (zolpidem) or Lunesta (eszopiclone) may be helpful.

Conclusion

Estrogen is not the enemy of women migraine sufferers. Estrogen is a natural part of who we are as women. Understanding the relationship between our hormones and migraines can be helpful as we work to develop effective treatment strategies. My hope is that this chapter can help you work with your healthcare provider to develop effective treatments for your hormonally related migraines. I also hope you now feel more empowered to make good choices for yourself in regards to hormone treatment.

Finally, I would like to end this chapter with a poem that has inspired me. It captures the "essence" of a woman "coming into her own" as she transitions in life to caring about what is important to her. I encourage you to listen to that quiet voice within and grow into your potential.

> **BOX 6-5   Second Spring**
>
> After a lifetime of caring for others
> As a working woman, wife or mother
> Meeting each new demand and then another
> Until it felt like I might smother
> Life has quieted down.
> Now I hear a voice, small and new,
> That says to me, "You matter, too."
> And I stand taller when I hear that sound.
> That's the wisdom that appears
> At the end of the child-bearing years.
> The wisdom to see
> The importance of ME
> And a voice to make sure
> The world hears.
>
> *Author: Unknown*

References

1. Sommerville BW. The role of estradiol withdrawal in the etiology of menstrual migraine. Neurology. 1972; 22(4): 355–365.
2. Important safety information. OrthoEvra Web Site. Available at http://www.orthoevra.com.
3. Sulak PJ, Cressman BE, Waldrop E, et al. Extending the duration of active oral contraceptive pills to manage hormone withdrawal symptoms. Obstet Gynecol. 1997; 89(2): 179–183.
4. Sulak PJ, Willis S, Kuehl T, et al. Headaches and oral contraceptives: impact of eliminating the standard 7-day placebo interval. Headache. 2007; 47: 27–37.

5. Pradalier A, Vincent D, Beaulieu PH, et al. Correlation between oestradiol plasma level and therapeutic effect on menstrual migraine. In: Rose RC, ed. *New Advances in Headache Research*, 4th ed. London: Smith-Gordon; 1994: 129–132.

6. Smite MG, van der Meer YG, Pfeil JP, et al. Perimenstrual migraine: effect of Estraderm TTS and the value of contingent negative variation and exeroceptive temporalis muscle suppression test. Headache. 1994; 34: 103–106.

7. MacGregor A, Frith A, Ellis J, et al. Prevention of menstrual attacks of migraine: a double-blind placebo-controlled cross-over study. Neurology. 2006; 67: 2159–2163.

8. Calhoun AH. A novel specific prophylaxis for menstrual-associated migraine. South Med J. 2004; 97(9): 819–822.

9. Fettes I. Migraine in the menopause. Neurology. 1999; 53(4 suppl 1): S29–S33.

10. Loprinzi CL, Kugler JW, Sloan JA, et al. Venlafaxine in management of hot flashes in survivors of breast cancer: a randomized controlled trial. Lancet. 2000; 356: 2059–2063.

11. Loprinzi CL, Sloan JA, Perez EA, et al. Phase III evaluation of fluoxetine for treatment of hot flashes. J Clin Oncol. 2002; 20: 1578–1583.

12. Guttoso T Jr, Kurlan R, McDermott MP, et al. Gabapentin's effects on hot flashes in postmenopausal women: a randomized controlled trial. Obstet Gynecol. 2003; 101: 337–345.

13. Fettes I. Migraine in the menopause. Neurology. 1999; 53(4 suppl 1): S29–S33.

14. Rossouw JE, Anderson GL, Prentice RL, et al., Risks and benefits of estrogen plus progestin in healthy postmenopausal women: principal results from the WHI randomized controlled trial. JAMA. 2002; 288(3): 321–333.

15. The 2012 Hormone Therapy Position Statement of The North American Menopause Society. Menopause: The Journal of the North American Menopause Society. 2012;19 (3): 257–271. Accessed www.menopause.org publications 11/04/12.

16. American College of Obstetrics and Gynecology (ACOG). *Guidelines for Women's Health Care: A Resource Manual*, 3rd ed., developed by the Editorial Committee for Guidelines for Women's Health Care (2003–2007). ACOG.

17. Nappi RE, Cagnacci A, Granella F, et al. Course of primary headaches during hormone replacement therapy. Maturitas. 2001; 38: 157–163.

7

Nonpharmacologic Treatment of Migraine in Women

Nancy, 29, is frustrated. As an attorney, she needs to be alert and focused at all times. Some of the migraine preventive medications she has tried make her too sleepy during the day; others have made her anxious and agitated. She asks, "What can I take that is more natural? Are there any herbs that can help my headaches? A friend of mine told me to take feverfew."

❖

Melanie, 35, is frustrated. She has been diagnosed as having depression and fibromyalgia in addition to menstrual migraines. She does not want to keep taking prescription medications. She asks, "What else can I do to help my migraines, depression, and fibromyalgia? A friend of mine recommended acupuncture."

❖

In this chapter, we will try to answer the questions that Nancy and Melanie raise. You may already be thinking of other alternative nonprescription treatments for your migraines. But which treatments have the best chance of success? We look at what the research supports and review the following areas of nonpharmacologic treatment

- Herbal and homeopathic products
- Biofeedback
- Cognitive-behavioral therapy (CBT)
- Relaxation exercises
- Stress management
- Physical therapy
- Massage therapy
- Acupuncture
- Chiropractic
- Exercise
- Sleep
- Diet
- Other strategies

Herbal Products

Herbal products have been used for migraine prevention for years, but some are better studied than others. The following are those herbal compounds that I feel are most useful for migraine prevention, including menstrual migraine:

- Magnesium: 400 mg total daily dose (usually 200 mg twice a day)
- Riboflavin (vitamin B$_2$): 400 mg total daily dose
- Petadolex (butterbur): 75 mg twice a day

Possibly effective:

- Feverfew
- Coenzyme Q-10: 150 mg twice a day

Most of these listed herbal products will be effective without causing uncomfortable side effects, although magnesium may cause diarrhea in some individuals. Many of the products can be found in combination, in products such as Migrelief (magnesium, feverfew, and B$_2$) and Trigemin (same ingredients as Migrelief with additional products for optimal brain health). To learn more go to www.migrelief.com or www.trigemin.com.

Magnesium has been well-studied in the prevention of menstrual migraine. One double-blind study showed that magnesium pyrrolidone carboxylic acid (360 mg a day), when taken during the second half of the menstrual cycle, decreased the duration and severity of menstrual migraine compared to the placebo group.[1] Most of my patients with menstrual migraine find it easier to simply take magnesium every day of their cycle, and the majority of them take it in the form of an over-the-counter combination tablet called Migrelief. If diarrhea is a problem, then sometimes lowering the dose or switching to a different form of magnesium can be helpful.

Petadolex (butterbur) has been shown to be effective in a number of clinical trials. In a multicenter, placebo-controlled, double-blind study of 245 patients, 71% responded to treatment at 75 mg twice a day, whereas 60% responded to treatment at 50 mg twice a day.[2] Looking at all patients taking Petadolex in this study, investigators found 58% fewer migraine attacks.[2] In a smaller study of 60 patients, there was a 55% reduction in the need to use acute therapy in patients taking 75 mg twice a day.[3]

Vitamin B$_2$ is riboflavin, one of the B vitamins. It is water soluble and can be safely taken by pregnant and breastfeeding women for migraine prevention. It is very well-tolerated, inexpensive, and has been used at headache centers for many years. Published studies demonstrate that high-dose riboflavin (400 mg a day) decreases both the frequency and intensity of migraine.[4]

These results are significant because acute medications like triptans can get expensive, and patients are often afraid they are going to run out of their insurance-allocated number of pills when they most need them. Most patients tolerate Petadolex well, although it should not be used during pregnancy or breastfeeding or in patients with liver disease. There are other sources of butterbur, but the Petadolex brand has been shown effective in clinical studies, and there is no guarantee that other brands will be as effective. For that reason, I usually recommend that my patients take the Petadolex brand of butterbur.

For Nancy, our frustrated attorney, I recommended a regimen consisting of 75 mg of Petadolex twice a day plus 1 Migrelief tablet twice a day. When using herbal therapy for prevention of migraine, I advise women to give a new therapy a full 3 months before deciding if the treatment is effective. Herbal remedies often take longer to reach full benefit but, compared with many prescription medications, they are easier to tolerate and are much less expensive.

Homeopathic Products

For acute migraine relief, I have had patients report success with a Hyland's Homeopathic Product called Migraine Headache Relief.[5] One of my patients rarely needs her Maxalt (rizatriptan) because she takes Migraine Headache Relief instead. This is strictly an anecdotal report and not backed up by scientific studies. Homeopathic products are considered "alternative" medical preparations.

Biofeedback

Biofeedback, a shortened way of saying "biological feedback," shows individuals what is going on in their bodies. Administered by psychologists, it is a treatment that involves monitoring and bringing under control involuntary physiological functions such as muscle tension, finger temperature, or blood pressure. Control of these functions can reduce migraine.

There are different types of biofeedback, including thermal (which monitors the warmth of the hand; sometimes called "hand warming") and electromyography (EMG), which monitors muscle response. Thermal biofeedback appears to be the most effective for migraine prevention, and EMG is most effective for tension-type headache prevention. In thermal biofeedback, a patient is connected to a biofeedback machine that measures finger temperature. This information is converted to a signal that is presented to the patient; the patient is then taught to raise his or her finger temperature. This raising of the finger temperature causes a more relaxed state in the body, which can help migraine. Over a period of time, the individual can raise her finger temperature without needing the biofeedback machine. For EMG biofeedback, the biofeedback machine measures muscle tension, usually in the head or neck. The goal is to learn to lower tension in those muscles that are often tensed and contribute to both tension and migraine headaches. Biofeedback requires a series of sessions, often 6 to 12. Not all psychologists are trained in biofeedback, so it is important to ask before being referred by your primary care provider. See these two websites for more information and to find a certified biofeedback provider:www.bcia.org/directory/membership.cfm and www.aapb.org. For self-training biofeedback, see www.headachecare.com (you can obtain a biofeedback kit, including a finger thermometer).

Cognitive-Behavioral Therapy

Cognitive-behavioral therapy differs from traditional "psychotherapy" or counseling. CBT focuses on negative thinking and negative behaviors, with the goal of reversing negative thoughts and actions to positive, affirmative thinking and better behavior, including lifestyle. CBT has been considered effective in migraine prevention according to U.S. Headache Consortium Guidelines, and it is often combined with biofeedback, relaxation training, and stress management. Specific aspects of CBT may include challenging feelings of hopelessness, increasing coping skills, assertiveness training, and improved self-esteem. If a migraine sufferer is coping better in life, has better self-esteem, and takes more responsibility for her attitude and lifestyle, her migraines will be under better control. Nancy, the 29-year-old attorney, for example, feels as if there is little she can do to control her migraines; rather, she feels they control her. With CBT, she can take more responsibility for her migraines, including being more in charge of avoiding triggers and practicing a healthy lifestyle. Over time, she can start to feel that she is living her life in spite of her migraines.

Thirty-five-year old Melanie is feeling very overwhelmed with her recent diagnosis of fibromyalgia and has been feeling incapable of managing her health. Melanie would be an excellent candidate for CBT because it has been shown helpful in treating depression and fibromyalgia, disorders she suffers from, in addition to anxiety, panic attacks, obsessive-compulsive disorder, and sleep disorders. Since Melanie also suffers from depression, I would recommend that she combine CBT with prescription medication and attention to lifestyle for maximum improvement in quality of life. With CBT, Melanie can feel empowered to take charge of her life and live life in spite of her medical conditions.

A first step toward wellness is confronting the negative thinking or beliefs that hold you back. Do you play the victim role or get stuck in a negative cycle of thinking that your migraines will never get better? Do you get stuck in bad habits such as drinking too much alcohol, not exercising, binge eating, under- or oversleeping, or skipping meals? CBT may be useful for you. Not all therapists and psychologists are trained in CBT. To learn more, go to the Association for Behavioral and Cognitive Therapies web site at www.aabt.org.

Relaxation Exercises

Lisa, the 25-year-old teacher, feels stressed trying to cope with the demands of teaching, her migraines, and her marriage. Her neck muscles are tight, and sometimes it hurts to even turn her head. Lately, she feels it is impossible for her to relax as she is always worried about something and can't "let it go." She complains "I don't have time to get to the gym; I have too much to do with my class including lesson plans, calling parents, and grading papers. Sometimes I wonder if it was a mistake to become a teacher."

Relaxation techniques could make a real difference in Lisa's life and could help her better manage her stress, tight muscles, and migraines. Specific relaxation training often includes breathing exercises, meditation, exercises to relax the muscles in the neck and shoulders, yoga, self-hypnosis, prayer, and listening to relaxation tapes (including music geared at calming the mind and body). Relaxation techniques can be self-taught through CDs, tapes, websites, and books but are often best learned through trained professionals, usually psychologists or therapists. To be effective in managing migraine, as well as associated conditions such as tight muscles and anxiety, these relaxation exercises should be practiced daily.

Stress Management

Stress is a known trigger for migraine headaches. Along with hormones, stress is the most common migraine trigger for my patients. Stress, unfortunately, is a part of life. Although we cannot prevent stressful events in our lives, we can control our reactions to those stressful events. CBT, relaxation exercises, and biofeedback can help teach a migraine sufferer to better handle stress. There are also many "easy" activities that we can include in our lives to help with stress. Physical exercise, engaging in pleasurable activities such as reading a book or going to a movie, spending time with a friend, sexual activity, having a massage, and engaging in a pleasurable hobby can all be stress-reducers and help give us the balance in life that we all need.

Take Nancy. She has a high-stress job, frequent migraines, a hectic work schedule, irritable bowel syndrome, and a history of emotional and physical abuse. She joined a high-end gym near her work and now goes there three or four times a week after work and on the weekends. She is taking a yoga class, does weight-training, and some cardio on the elliptical machine, and is feeling less stressed. She has also met a few nice women at the gym and now looks forward to her time there. She tells me that a wonderful feeling of euphoria and well-being comes over her at the end of her workout, and that feeling stays with her during her drive home from the gym. She is feeling less hopeless about her migraines and her life in general.

BOX 7-1

Learn what activities and hobbies reduce your stress. Practice them regularly. You will feel more in charge of your life, and your migraines will improve.

All the women migraine sufferers we have met in this book need to practice stress-reduction. Take Lisa, who feels anxious and unable to relax, and complains she has no time for herself. She needs to *make* time for herself, even if that means saying no to others. Saying no to others can mean saying yes to you.

Physical Therapy

Physical therapy can significantly improve headache and neck pain in many women suffering from migraine. The initial physical therapy assessment may include evaluating those muscle areas of tightness and pain that are contributing to or causing the headache. Attention to proper posture, stretching exercises, and correction of day-to-day activities that are aggravating the pain can all be evaluated. Many of us spend hours in front of a computer, ignoring good posture, and we end up with a lot of neck and back pain. Others are lifting and carrying groceries, kids, and heavy purses or backpacks, not realizing how some of those activities can be aggravating neck and back pain.

An advantage of physical therapy over some of the other treatments mentioned in this chapter is that it is usually a covered benefit under medical insurance plans. I recommend everyone with neck pain, back pain, and frequent headaches (migraine or tension) to go for a physical therapy evaluation.

Usually, physical therapy will involve 2–3 visits a week for 4–6 weeks; then, the patient will transition to doing stretching exercises and home treatment as instructed by the physical therapist. When appropriate, home physical therapy equipment such as traction units or transcutaneous electrical stimulation (TENS) units may be arranged for home use.

Massage Therapy

Massage therapy can be very helpful in relaxing the mind as well as tight muscles. There are many different types of massage, including traditional Swedish massage, deeper tissue sports-type massage, and more.

Usually, massage is not covered by medical insurance so it can become expensive if done regularly to prevent migraine. Often, targeted massage of specific tight muscles can be done as part of physical therapy, and this form of treatment would have better insurance coverage.

Acupuncture

Acupuncture therapy involves the placement of small needles in specific points on the body that are believed to correlate with certain painful areas. The needles can stimulate endorphin release, which can help with migraine reduction. Endorphins are naturally produced peptides that cause a feeling of euphoria (feeling good or "high"). Studies of acupuncture have had difficulty showing benefit over the "sham" or placebo group but, overall, there appears to be a trend showing acupuncture to be beneficial.[6] In my practice, I have had many women migraine patients believe that acupuncture was beneficial, including during pregnancy. Acupuncture can help during a migraine headache attack and can also help with prevention.

Chiropractic Treatment

The type of treatment provided by chiropractors can vary from "cracking" or "adjusting" someone's neck or back to physical therapy modalities such as stretching, traction, and electrical stimulation. In my practice, once I get a good history from my migraine patients, I often find overlap in what is provided by physical therapy and chiropractors. The bottom line for my patients is that the treatment is beneficial and does not hurt or aggravate them. I have found that referring a migraine patient to a chiropractor is especially beneficial when there is neck pain in addition to the headaches.

Exercise

Regular exercise should be part of everyone's lifestyle but especially for women migraine sufferers since exercise has been found to decrease the frequency of migraine in clinical studies. Exercise can also reduce stress and help with sleep, and improved sleep often helps prevent migraine.

Sleep

Sleep is crucial for everyone, but sleep complaints are common among migraine sufferers. In a large survey study of more than 1,000 migraine patients, 31% reported trouble in falling asleep and 30% reported trouble staying asleep.[7] In this same study, patients sleeping 6 hours or less each night reported more frequent and severe headaches than did those sleeping 6–8 hours a night. Those who slept longer, more than 8 hours, also reported greater headache activity.[6] Many other studies support the relationship between disturbed sleep and more frequent or severe headaches.

Many migraine sufferers report that their migraine attacks jolt them awake in the middle of the night or they wake up with a full-blown migraine. One study found that 42% of patients reported that more than 75% of their migraines occurred either at night or between 3 a.m. and 7 a.m.[8] The link between migraine and sleep is thought to occur because of changes in serotonin, melatonin, and magnesium levels. We don't know the exact relationship yet, but it may have to do with serotonin from the pineal gland in the brain being converted or changed to melatonin. Elevated serotonin levels from the pineal gland and reduced melatonin levels may increase headache activity.[9] In a study that compared plasma melatonin levels in those who suffer from migraine with those the same age who do not, lower plasma melatonin levels were seen in migraine sufferers.[10] In another study, lower levels of magnesium in body cells were seen in college students in a sleep deprivation study compared to levels in the students at baseline.[11]

I recommend that migraine sufferers try to get consistently 7–8 hours of sleep every night. Ideally, a person suffering with migraines should go to bed at the same time every evening and get up at the same time every morning.

Melatonin also helps. In a small study, researchers reported that taking 3 mg of melatonin 30 minutes before bedtime for 3 months reduced the number of migraines by 61%.[12] Some individuals may prefer an extended-release form of melatonin (melatonin ER) if they have trouble staying asleep. In my opinion, melatonin is a safe addition to other preventive treatments that a patient may be taking.

If the simple measures discussed here are not helpful in improving sleep, then a more complete sleep evaluation may be needed, including an overnight sleep study to look for problems such as sleep apnea (disruption in breathing during sleep).

More research is needed to better understand the relationship between sleep and migraine activity. In the meantime, these are my recommendations:

- Get between 7–8 hours of good-quality sleep.
- Establish consistent sleep habits by going to bed at the same time and getting up at the same time, even on weekends.
- Supplement with melatonin 3 mg at night if you are experiencing trouble getting to sleep.
- Consider supplementing with 400 mg of magnesium a day, which may also help prevent migraines that are related to sleep.

Diet

Nancy often skips breakfast or lunch when she has a busy schedule. When she begins to get hungry, she eats but then complains that it's too late—her migraine gets worse even though she stops to eat. Her problem is that she's not eating at regular times. Women with migraine ideally should never skip meals and should try to eat at approximately the same times every day. Meals should be balanced, with adequate protein at each meal since protein can slow down the absorption of carbohydrates and help to keep blood sugar levels even: Fluctuations in blood sugar can trigger a migraine.

Not everyone has food triggers for migraines. As a result, I don't put all of my migraine patients on strict diets. If they're keeping headache diaries, as I recommend for *all* migraine sufferers, then they will be able to see if certain foods or additives trigger migraine attacks. I often ask patients to recall what they were eating or drinking for the 24 hours leading up to a particular attack and then to look for patterns; most are able to figure out their food triggers within a few months. Common migraine triggers include:

- Monosodium glutamate (MSG)
- Nitrates
- Aspartame (artificial sweetener)
- NutraSweet (artificial sweetener)
- Alcohol
- Caffeine

- Cheese (especially aged cheese)
- Nuts
- Chocolate
- Gluten

These websites are useful for anyone seeking more information on dietary triggers for migraine: www.achenet.org and www.headaches.org.

Less Common Treatments

Other treatment that doesn't involve medication may include *oral devices and correction of problems in the mouth or jaw* (e.g., temporal mandibular joint problems [TMJ]). If you have pain in your jaw and are either unable to open up your jaw completely or without pain, then I recommend evaluation with an orofacial pain specialist. Usually, orofacial pain specialists are dentists who have completed specialized training and are better able to handle complicated issues involving the mouth, teeth, and jaw.

Another new treatment that may help with migraine prevention is *transcranial magnetic stimulation* (TMS). Currently, TMS is only FDA-approved for resistant depression, but it also shows promise for migraine prevention. It is noninvasive but requires multiple treatments, 5 days a week for about 6 weeks; at this time, is cost-prohibitive for most patients.

Trigger point injections with a topical anesthetic or numbing medication, such as lidocaine or bupivacaine, can be helpful in relieving tight muscles that are contributing to neck pain and migraines. These injections often give immediate relief but results usually wear off after 2 weeks. In some cases, the anesthetic is combined with a steroid to produce longer lasting benefit. If I have patients receiving trigger point injections, I also like them to see a physical therapist who can work with them on reducing muscle tightness and teach them home exercises for prevention. In some cases, biofeedback with EMG may be beneficial.

Occipital nerve blocks can be easily done as an outpatient procedure and involve using a small needle to inject a topical anesthetic (e.g., bupivacaine) into the greater occipital nerve in the back of the head area. The anesthetic is usually injected on both sides. It may be combined with a steroid. In my experience, occipital nerve blocks can bring immediate relief for those suffering from a prolonged migraine. However, the benefits often only last for 2 weeks.

Botox (botulinum toxin) is now FDA approved for migraine prevention. The recommended dose for chronic migraine prevention is 155 units. Botox can help prevent migraines and chronic headache for 3 months in most cases. In my practice, Botox is usually offered to migraine patients who have failed traditional preventive treatment such as oral Topamax (topiramate).

Creating Your Own Wellness Plan

For myself, stress was one of the biggest barriers to overcoming my migraine problem. Years ago, I remember complaining to a friend that I simply could not find the time for a regular exercise program. Between my clinical practice, involvement in professional associations, and family commitments, I had started to feel run down, like everyone wanted a "piece of me." I felt as if there wasn't anything left over for "me."

My friend sagely replied, "No one else will give you the time to exercise. You have to *take* that time." His words had a great impact on me. In an informal way, he was practicing CBT, in that he brought my attention to the way I think and behave.

To this day, Monday and Wednesday evenings are "my nights" at the gym. I am in a Masters Swim Class and do my best to never miss a class. When I am asked to do other activities on those evenings, I simply reply "That's my gym night; I try to not let anything get in the way of that." It is empowering to carve time out for yourself and consider it as important as an appointment or a date with a friend.

Another simple strategy is one I learned from my own therapist, who I was seeing to help manage my stress. The therapist assigned me the task of writing down 10 activities that made me happy. I wrote down activities like going for a walk on the beach, making chocolate chip cookies, playing the piano, sleeping in and enjoying that first cup of coffee in bed, going out to dinner and a movie with a girlfriend, and going for a swim. She then assigned me the task of doing as many of those activities as I could before I saw her again in several weeks. This was terrific homework for me since I had never given myself enough of my own attention, and I felt immediately less stressed. Since then, I have learned to occasionally stop and write down a list of what is important to me and what I want to do and accomplish. Not only has this helped me stay in tune with my own goals, but it has helped me manage my migraines.

What do you need to say no to? What activities or hobbies do you need to say yes to?

Conclusion

Women suffering with migraine should seek to incorporate lifestyle changes along with their medications to create an overall migraine management plan. Those who do will achieve better quality of life than will those who only rely on prescription medications for their migraine attacks. I encourage you to exercise regularly; eat healthy, balanced meals; get good-quality sleep; and be aware of other alternative treatments that may be helpful for you. I hope this chapter will help you develop an effective migraine management plan that helps lessen the burden of migraine, including menstrual migraine, in your life.

References

1. Facchinetti F, Sances G, Borella P, et al. Magnesium prophylaxis of menstrual migraine: effects on intracellular magnesium. Headache. 1991; 31: 298–301.

2. Lipton RB, et al. Multi-center, placebo-controlled, double-blind study with 245 patients in accordance with the International Headache Society criteria. Neurology. 2004; 63: 2240–2244.

3. Diener HC, Rahlfs VW, Danesch U. The first placebo-controlled trial of a special butterbur root extract for the prevention of migraine: reanalysis of efficacy criteria. Eur Neurol. 2004: 51: 89–97.

4. Schoenen J, Jacquy J, Lenaerts M. Effectiveness of high-dose riboflavin in migraine prophylaxis: a randomized controlled trial. Neurology. 1998; 50: 466–470.

5. www.hyland's.com. Accessed September 19, 2010.

6. Melchart D, Linde K, Fischer P, et al. Acupuncture for recurrent headaches: a systematic review of randomized controlled trials. Cephalalgia. 1999; 19: 779–786.

7. Kelman L, Rains JC. Headache and sleep: examination of sleep patterns and complaints in a large clinical sample of migraineurs. Headache. 2005; 45: 904–910.

8. Gori S, Morelli N, Maestri M, et al. Sleep quality, chronotypes and preferential timing of attacks in migraine without aura. J Headache Pain. 2005; 6: 258–260.

9. Toglia JU. Melatonin: a significant contributor to the pathogenesis of migraine. Med Hypotheses. 2001: 57: 432–434.

10. Claustrat B, Loisy C, Brun J, et al. Nocturnal plasma melatonin levels in migraine: a preliminary report. Headache. 1989; 29: 242–245.

11. Takase B, Akima T, Satomura K, et al Effects of chronic sleep deprivation on autonomic activity by examining heart rate variability, plasma catecholamine, and intracellular magnesium levels. Biomed Pharamacother. 2004; 58(suppl 1): S35–S39.

12. Peres MP, Zukerman E, da Cunha Tanuri F, et al. Melatonin, 3 mg, is effective for migraine prevention. Neurology. 2004; 63: 757.

8

Pregnancy and Breastfeeding

> *Lisa, the 25-year-old teacher we met in Chapter 1, has endometriosis in addition to her menstrual migraines. She is hoping to get pregnant within the next year and has been told that getting pregnant would help her endometriosis. However, she is taking a lot of Excedrin (acetaminophen-aspirin-caffeine combination) and Imitrex (sumatriptan) for her migraines and is worried about taking medications during pregnancy. She currently is on a continuous low-dose birth control pill to suppress endometriosis. She also suffers from anxiety, and her doctor recommended she go on Lexapro (escitalopram). However, she doesn't know if Lexapro would be safe during pregnancy and is hesitant to start taking it. Understandably, Lisa is very stressed about everything!*

What can we tell Lisa about migraines, including treatment options, during pregnancy and breastfeeding?

Migraine peaks in women during their child-bearing years. With as many as 50% of pregnancies unplanned, the choice of migraine medications needs to take into account safety issues during pregnancy. Many women don't want to take any prescription medication during pregnancy for fear it will affect their fetuses. But untreated migraine attacks during pregnancy can be complicated by vomiting, potential dehydration, and disabling pain. It may be better, in many cases, to take medication to treat the attack than to suffer and risk dehydration and the other negative consequences of an untreated migraine attack.

Fortunately, we can reassure Lisa and others like her that most women will experience improvement in their migraines during pregnancy. In fact, a major study showed that almost 75% of women who have migraine without aura report improvement in headaches during pregnancy,[1] and, in a clinical review of a large number of studies involving migraine and pregnancy, women experiences a 60–70% improvement in migraine during pregnancy; in approximately 20% of these women, migraine attacks completely disappeared during pregnancy.[2]

Estrogen is the cause of this improvement. As discussed in Chapter 6, the drop in estrogen before menstruation is considered the strongest trigger for menstrual migraine. During pregnancy, estrogen levels rise and then stay level or steady until delivery. This high, steady level of estrogen is believed to be the main reason that many women report major improvement in their migraines during pregnancy. A woman with a history of menstrual migraine will likely do better during pregnancy than her friend whose migraines have no association with menstruation. Therefore, we can reassure Lisa that there is a very good chance her migraines will improve or go away during pregnancy.

Unfortunately, not all women experience improvement in their migraines during pregnancy. If headaches are not improved by the end of the first trimester (the first 12 weeks), then they are unlikely to improve during the second and third trimesters.[3] Also, those women who have migraine with aura do not show as much improvement; in fact, the higher levels of estrogen during pregnancy may actually aggravate aura.[4]

Some women—about 7%—will experience migraine for the first time during pregnancy.[5] These women are likely to have aura with their new-onset migraine attacks.[6] Researchers believe that the high levels of estrogen during pregnancy are responsible for aura in these cases.

Planning for Pregnancy

Lisa is reassured and optimistic that her migraines may go away or get better during migraines—but she still has a lot of questions as she considers going off her birth control pills in 6 months to begin trying to get pregnant. She asks, "What should I do now as I plan ahead for a pregnancy?"

To start, Lisa should be instructed to begin taking folic acid to reduce the risk of her baby having a neural tube defect. All women of child-bearing years, not just those with migraine, are advised to taken a multivitamin containing at least 0.4 mg (400 micrograms [mcg]) of folic acid daily. Folic acid is often added to enriched grain products such as breads, cereals, and pasta but, for most women, eating these foods would still not give them the recommended daily amount of folic acid.

During pre-pregnancy planning, I encourage women to review the following issues with their physicians:

- Prescription medications
- Herbal supplements, homeopathic medications, and over-the-counter medication use
- Lifestyle, including diet

Prescription Medications and Pre-pregnancy

In general, the use of daily preventive migraine medications should be discontinued if possible. If this is not possible, then using the lowest effective dose of the preventive is advisable. Fewer than 30 drugs have been proven to be harmful to the fetus at normally prescribed doses.[7] Therefore, if women are taking medications in the early weeks of pregnancy, before they know they are pregnant, it is not necessary to terminate the pregnancy in most cases. Common migraine preventives that should be stopped before attempting pregnancy include:

- Depakote (divalproex sodium)
- Topamax (topiramate)
- Methysergide
- Lisinopril
- Candesartan
- Paxil (paroxetine)
- Herbal and homeopathic preventives (with the exception of magnesium and vitamin B_2, which are probably safe during pregnancy)

Topamax (topiramate), until early March 2011, was considered fairly safe for use during pregnancy. However, the U.S. Food and Drug Administration (FDA) has changed its guidelines due to data that suggested an increased risk for the development of cleft lip and/or cleft palate in infants born to women treated with Topamax during pregnancy.

Medications to avoid during pre-pregnancy for treating conditions other than migraine include:

- Coumadin (warfarin)
- Tegretol (carbamazepine)
- Dilantin (phenytoin)
- Retin A (isotretinoin)
- Cholesterol-lowering medications
- Blue cohosh
- Yellow ginseng
- Cytotec (misoprostol)

- Ribavirin
- Interferon-a[8]

Acute migraine attack medications that should be avoided during pregnancy planning include:

- Cafergot (ergotamine-caffeine)
- Ergostat (ergotamine)
- Migranal nasal spray (dihydroergotamine)
- Dihydroergotamine (DHE)

The use of nonmedication treatments for migraine prevention during pregnancy can be very useful during prepregnancy, as such treatments may help women wean off some of their prescription preventives. Effective treatments may include biofeedback, relaxation exercises, stress-reduction measures, physical therapy, and acupuncture. See Chapter 7 for more details on nonpharmacologic migraine treatments.

The Effect of Migraine on Pregnancy

Lisa read on the Internet that migraine might increase her risk of complications during pregnancy. She wonders what her risks are, given her history as a migraine sufferer. Many studies suggest that women with migraine have a higher risk of preeclampsia and eclampsia than do women without migraine; this risk is even higher in women who were 30 years or older when they were diagnosed with migraine and in overweight women.[9] Preeclampsia is characterized by high blood pressure, fluid retention, and protein in the urine; it is associated with an increased risk of stroke, seizures, and placental abruption (separation of the placenta from the uterus).

Migraine is also a risk factor for developing *gestational hypertension*, or elevated blood pressure during pregnancy, and pregnancy-related stroke. Risk of stroke increases with age and is highest in women older than 35 years.

Luckily, studies do not show an increased risk of birth defects or other problems in babies born to mothers with migraine.

Treatment of Migraine During Pregnancy

The good news for most women with migraine is that their migraines will most likely go away or improve during pregnancy. During pregnancy, estrogen levels rise and then remain fairly steady until the time of delivery. The high, sustained level of estrogen is thought to be the main reason for migraine improvement during pregnancy; however, some migraine sufferers will still have migraines during pregnancy and, for some women, pregnancy will be the first time they experience migraine headaches.

So, which medications are safe for women to take during pregnancy? Unfortunately, the American College of Obstetrics and Gynecology (ACOG) has not yet provided established guidelines, and obstetricians vary in what they allow their pregnant patients to take. Most want their pregnant patients to avoid taking any medications for headache during pregnancy, but that may not be possible for women suffering from moderate to severe migraine headaches.

I encourage my patients to become familiar with the FDA pregnancy risk rating system, since most healthcare providers use it to help make treatment decisions. The FDA assigns medication into five categories as follows:

- Category A: Controlled human studies show no risk to the fetus
- Category B: No evidence of risk in humans but with no controlled human studies
- Category C: Risk to humans has "not been ruled out"
- Category D: Positive evidence of risk from human or animal studies
- Category X: Pregnancy risk is so definite that the drug is absolutely advised against during pregnancy

In general, the safest medication to take for migraine attacks during pregnancy are those with a Category A or B rating. These include:

- Tylenol (acetaminophen)
- Caffeine
- Antinausea medications:
  - Zofran (ondansetron)
  - Reglan (metoclopramide)
- Periactin (cyproheptadine, an antihistamine)

Many obstetricians will prescribe a class of pain medication called opioids if migraine attacks are severe during pregnancy. Opioids include Vicodin (hydrocodone), codeine (e.g., Tylenol with codeine), and Demerol (meperidine).

Anti-Inflammatory Medication

Opioids should be used sparingly for the treatment of migraine during pregnancy since opioid dependency can be passed from mother to infant. If it is completely necessary, limiting the amount of medication taken will help prevent withdrawal symptoms in the infant.

Anti-inflammatory medications such as aspirin, Aleve (naproxen), and Motrin (ibuprofen) are generally not recommended during pregnancy. Some obstetricians allow pregnant patients to take Aleve or Motrin at the beginning of the pregnancy, but most recommend complete avoidance. Most of the anti-inflammatory medications are pregnancy Category C for the first and second trimesters, then are elevated to Category D for the third trimester. There have been some reports of an increased risk of miscarriage if nonsteroidal anti-inflammatory drugs (NSAIDs) are used in early pregnancy;[10] however, in the third trimester, it is critical to completely avoid anti-inflammatory medications. One of the more dire risks includes the premature closing of the ductus arteriosus, a blood vessel in the developing fetus.

Triptans

The triptan class of migraine medication is considered Category C, along with the majority of migraine medications classified including codeine, butalbital, and hydrocodone. Since triptans were introduced into the U.S. market in 1993, with Imitrex (sumatriptan) the first available, many migraine sufferers regularly use triptans for treatment of acute migraine attacks. There are now seven different triptans and, fortunately, there does not appear to be an increased risk of complications during pregnancy associated with their use. Since Imitrex has been on the market the longest of its class, we have the benefit of plentiful data in the pregnancy database registry for this drug.

Pregnancy database registries are collections of cases reported by women who take a medication when they are pregnant. Often, this medication use occurs in the early weeks of pregnancy, before a woman knows she is pregnant. At other times, a physician may decide to allow a woman to take a medication during pregnancy because the benefit is felt to outweigh the risk of the medication. If a woman's case is reported by her healthcare provider to the registry, she will be followed throughout her pregnancy and will be watched for any problems, such as miscarriage, complications, or problems with the baby at delivery. Then, any complications that arise will be compared with the experiences of women who have not taken that particular medication. The benefits to this system are obvious: Physicians sharing information about their patients will lead to more data, which will help other physicians help future mothers-to-be make better decisions.

For example, as of October 31, 2010, there were 602 pregnancy outcomes from 594 pregnancy cases (including six sets of twins and one set of triplets) in the Imitrex (sumatriptan) registry of women who took Imitrex during pregnancy. The Registry Advisory Committee concluded that there was no evidence to suggest teratogenicity (congenital defects) in the infant from sumatriptan use by the mother.[11] However, the numbers are still too small to reach definitive conclusions. The Sumatriptan Registry is now closed since the reassuring data are supported by much larger datasets. A published study reported on 69,929 pregnant women and their newborns in Norway and concluded there is no association between triptan therapy during the first trimester and major congenital abnormalities, although there was a slight increase in atonic uterus and bleeding at the time of delivery when a triptan was taken during the second and third trimesters.[12] The Swedish Medical Birth Registry collects data on nearly all births (more than 95%) in Sweden. A total of 658 women who had used sumatriptan in pregnancy were reviewed in a published study in 2010. There appeared to be no difference in the rate of congenital malformations seen in infants exposed to sumatriptan compared to the prevalence seen in the general population of infants born.[13]

Some obstetricians are now comfortable with pregnant women using the triptans, such as Imitrex, during pregnancy; others tend to use older medications that they're more comfortable with, for example, narcotics and opioids including Vicodin (hydrocodone) and Tylenol (acetaminophen) with codeine. In a perfect world, pregnant women would not take any prescription medication for migraine attacks; however, we know that that is not realistic for moderate to severe attacks. It is not fair to women—and especially pregnant women—to suffer unnecessarily.

Treatment for Migraine Attacks

Lisa is in the exam room with her obstetrician and wants specific answers on how to treat her migraines during pregnancy. Her doctor recommends Tylenol (acetaminophen) for mild migraine attacks. For moderate attacks, he recommends one of the antinausea medications, such as Zofran (ondansetron) or Phenergan (promethazine). "But how will an antinausea medication help my head pain?" she asks. "Aren't those just for the nausea?"

First, let's address the use of Tylenol (acetaminophen) for mild migraine attacks. Tylenol is considered safe for pregnancy, but ideally its use should be limited to a maximum of two to three times a week to avoid liver damage. This is true for nonpregnant women as well.

And, yes, antinausea medications can indeed help migraine as well as nausea. They include:

- Zofran (ondansetron)
- Reglan (metoclopramide)
- Phenergan (promethazine)
- Compazine (prochlorperazine)
- Tigan (trimethobenzamide)

My favorite antinausea medication to recommend for patients, pregnant or not, is Zofran (ondansetron), which can be combined with other medications such as Tylenol or a triptan. Zofran conveniently comes in an oral dissolving tablet and is usually given in 8 mg doses every 8 hours as needed for nausea and headache. Some antinausea medications, such as Phenergan (promethazine) and Compazine (prochlorperazine), are available in rectal suppository form, which can be very useful if the pregnant woman is vomiting during her migraine attack and is unable to keep down an oral medication. Emetrol, phosphorated carbohydrate liquid medication, is available over-the-counter and generally considered safe. Should you need to go to the emergency room, you can take antinausea medications intravenously or through an injection.

Another medication sometimes used for moderate to severe migraine attacks during pregnancy is Ultram (tramadol). It is considered a pain medication, but is not as strong or as addictive as Vicodin (hydrocodone). Ultram is Category C for pregnancy.

Acute migraine medications that should be avoided during pregnancy include the ergots, anti-inflammatory medications, butalbital (Fioricet, Fiorinal), and Midrin (isometheptene-dichlorphenazone-acetaminophen; a combination medication that includes a vasoconstrictor that is not good in pregnancy). Some doctors may allow occasional use of Fioricet (butalbital-acetaminophen) during pregnancy but the butalbital can cause withdrawal problems in the infant if

TABLE 8-1 Quick guide to safe medications for migraine attacks during pregnancy

Mild-Moderate Migraine Attack	Moderate to Severe Migraine Attack
Tylenol, caffeine, increase hydration	Triptans (Imitrex preferred due
Zofran ODT, Phenergan, Reglan	to longest safety record and the
or other antinausea medication	large numbers in pregnancy
(Tigan, Compazine)	database registry compared to
Biofeedback, acupuncture,	other triptans), Vicodin, Tylenol
relaxation exercises, ice packs,	with codeine, Ultram, any of
trigger point or nerve block	these may be combined with
injections with topical	Zofran ODT or other antinausea
anesthetic	medication
Limit acute medication to	Emergency treatment: IV antinausea
maximum of twice a week to	medications such as Reglan or
prevent rebound.	Zofran, IV or injectable Demerol,
	IV magnesium, injectable Imitrex

taken late in pregnancy or close to delivery. In my opinion, Imitrex (sumatriptan) would be better than butalbital or narcotics taken late in pregnancy.

Table 8-1 shows, at a quick glance, the medications that I consider reasonable and safe during pregnancy.

Preventive Medication

Lisa is hopeful that her migraines will improve during pregnancy and that she won't have to consider a daily preventive for migraines. But some women experience frequent enough migraines during pregnancy that a prescription daily preventive may be necessary. In general, the medications believed to be the most effective, with the safest profile during pregnancy, would be those with a Category C rating. These include Inderal (propanolol), metoprolol, Neurontin (gabapentin), Prozac (fluoxetine), Elavil (amitriptyline), and verapamil.

Beta-blockers, antiepileptics, and tricyclic antidepressants are the general categories for prevention. My top choices when a daily preventive is needed in a pregnant woman would include:

- Inderal Long-Acting (propanolol LA), labetalol, or metoprolol (both beta-blockers)
- Elavil (amitriptyline, an antidepressant]

The decision to go on a daily preventive during pregnancy is a big one, and risks need to be weighed against benefits. The decision should be made between the obstetrician and the pregnant patient; in some cases, it may be necessary for the general practice obstetrician to consult with a high-risk obstetrician or a headache specialist. In many cases, the preventive can be tapered off as the delivery date approaches to prevent any withdrawal problems on the part of the infant.

Nonpharmacologic treatment during pregnancy can be very useful for migraine prevention and should be the mainstay of treatment in pregnant women with frequent migraines. Nonpharmacologic treatment options include:

- Hydration (especially with water)
- Healthy lifestyle
- Biofeedback
- Cognitive behavioral therapy (CBT)
- Stress reduction
- Relaxation exercises
- Acupuncture
- Biofeedback
- Massage
- Vitamin B$_2$ (riboflavin, 400 mg daily)
- Magnesium (400 mg daily)

For a more complete description of these treatment options, refer to Chapter 7.

A combination of nonpharmacologic preventive treatment options may be necessary to provide optimal prevention. Significantly, some behavioral treatments can be as effective as prescription medication for migraine prevention during pregnancy. One study compared the use of Elavil (amitriptyline) with a stress-management program and found equal benefit in headache reduction.[14] Another study combined thermal biofeedback with relaxation exercises and showed a 50–79% reduction in headache in a group of pregnant women; the benefits persisted past delivery.[15]

Several patients in my practice have found acupuncture to be very helpful in migraine prevention during pregnancy; acupuncture may also be helpful for acute migraine treatment. Another patient gave up her daily caffeine during pregnancy but when she got a migraine, she would drink a caffeinated beverage and get headache relief. See Table 8-2 for a summary of migraine prevention during pregnancy.

With all the prescription preventives listed, the lowest effective dose should be used. When considering dietary or herbal supplements like B_2 and magnesium, women should consult with their obstetricians.

TABLE 8-2 Migraine prevention during pregnancy

Nonpharmacologic prevention	Pharmacologic Treatment
Biofeedback, stress reduction, relaxation exercises, cognitive behavioral therapy, avoid known triggers, healthy lifestyle	First line (top choices): Inderal LA, labetalol, metoprolol
Not proven, but may help: Acupuncture, vitamin B_2, magnesium	Second line: Elavil, Prozac
	Third line: Gabapentin, verapamil
If neck pain: Physical therapy, massage therapy	Ideally, all preventives should be tapered in the last few weeks of pregnancy to avoid complications at delivery.

Treatment of Migraine During Breastfeeding

Lisa is worried about what will happen to her migraines after she delivers and is breastfeeding. She has read about the many benefits of breastfeeding but is worried about medication that could pass into the breast milk and affect her infant. What can we tell her? What do we know about medication and mother's milk?

First, we can reassure Lisa that many women will have fewer headaches if they breastfeed as opposed to formula-feed. This may have something to do with lessened hormonal fluctuation in women who choose to breastfeed. Second, we can reassure Lisa that most medications that were taken prior to pregnancy can be resumed after delivery with little to no potential harm for breastfeeding. There is a big difference in medication risk to a developing fetus in the womb compared to a newborn who is exposed to medication through his or her mother's breast milk.

Many women will enjoy fewer migraines during pregnancy but find that migraines increase once they deliver due to the marked drop in estrogen that characterizes the postpartum period. However, with breastfeeding, ovulation is often suppressed, so migraines may be infrequent and mild until breastfeeding is stopped or decreased—at which time ovulation usually returns. With ovulation, the normal ups and downs of estrogen and progesterone return and, with them, the return of menstrual migraine.

In my practice, many patients are pleased that they can take an anti-inflammatory like Aleve (naproxen) or Motrin (ibuprofen) for their postpartum headaches and not need their triptan. Typically, however, as the months pass and the volume of breastfeeding decreases, the severity of the headaches worsen and women once again reach for their triptans for headache relief.

Fortunately, more guidelines and resources are available for migraine treatment during breastfeeding than for migraine treatment during pregnancy. The leading national organization for pediatrics, the American Academy of Pediatrics (AAP), has published a policy statement, "The Transfer of Drugs and Other Chemicals into Human Milk."[16] This set of guidelines does not classify drugs as "safe" or "unsafe," but it does categorize drugs and other agents into seven tables based on what is known about the effect of the drug or agent on the infant or on lactation, if known. The seven tables are listed in Box 8-1.

Box 8-1

Table 1: Cytotoxic Drugs That May Interfere with Cellular Metabolism of the Nursing Infant

Table 2: Drugs of Abuse for Which Adverse Effects on the Infant during Breastfeeding Have Been Reported

Table 3: Radioactive Compounds That Require Temporary Cessation of Breastfeeding

Table 4: Drugs for Which the Effect on Nursing Infants is Unknown but May Be of Concern

Table 5: Drugs That Have Been Associated with Significant Effects on Some Nursing Infants and Should Be Given to Nursing Mothers with Caution

Table 6: Maternal Medications Usually Compatible with Breastfeeding

Table 7: Food and Environmental Agents: Effects on Breastfeeding

The full policy statement can be viewed on the AAP website at http://aappolicy.aappublications.org/cgi/reprint/pediatrics;108/3/776.pdf.

Another useful and more practical reference is a textbook called *Medications and Mothers Milk* by Thomas Hale.[17] This textbook, updated frequently, is a thorough and comprehensive manual containing a complete review of what has been published about medications in breastfeeding mothers. I recommend this reference as an excellent resource for any woman who wants knowledge of medication choices at her fingertips. Dr. Hale has developed a lactation risk category rating that he applies to all the medications listed in the manual. These categories are outlined in Table 8-3.

TABLE 8-3 Hales Lactation Risk Categories. Adapted from *Medications and Mothers Milk*, Thomas Hale.

Lactation Risk Category 1: SAFEST: Drug has been taken by a large number of breastfeeding mothers without any observed adverse effect in the infant

Lactation Risk Category 2: SAFER: Drug has been studied in a limited number of breastfeeding women without an increase in adverse effects in the infant

Lactation Risk Category 3: MODERATELY SAFE: No controlled studies in breastfeeding women; however, the risk of untoward effects to a breastfed infant is possible; or, controlled studies show only minimal, nonthreatening adverse effects. (New medications that have no published data are automatically put in this category, regardless of how safe they are.)

Lactation Risk Category 4: POSSIBLY HAZARDOUS: Positive evidence of risk to a breastfed infant or to breast milk production, but benefits may be acceptable if the drug is needed for a serious condition of the mother

Lactation Risk Category 5: CONTRAINDICATED: Studies indicate significant and documented risk to the infant based on human experience, or it is a medication that has a high risk of causing significant damage to an infant.

Migraine medications listed in Lactation Categories 1 and 2 would be most desirable for women who are breastfeeding but need to treat migraine attacks. Lactation Category 3 would be acceptable in most cases. Specific medications and category ratings will be discussed later in this chapter.

Finally, a third useful source for medical information on drugs and breastfeeding is an online database available to anyone who wants more information when making decisions on medication safety for breastfeeding: http://toxnet.nlm.nih.gov/cgi-bin/sis/htmlgen?LACT

This free database[18] is part of the National Library of Medicine's TOXNET system and contains more than 450 drug records. It's easy to use. Go to the homepage and simply enter the name of the medication you want to learn more about (e.g., Naprosyn or Motrin), and all the information that is currently known about that medication in regards to breastfeeding will appear on the screen. The level of medication that seeps into the breast milk is discussed, as are the drug levels in the infant, any potential effects of the medication on breast-milk production, and, perhaps most important, any negative effects on the breastfeeding infant.

Having fluency and familiarity with these three resources when planning treatment will empower you to make the best possible decisions.

Medications for Migraine Attacks in Breastfeeding Women

Medications for acute migraine attacks fall into several categories, listed here. I'll address their effectiveness and safety in turn, highlighting the most popular formulations.

- Analgesics (pain relievers)
- Antiemetics (antinausea medications)
- Ergots and ergot alkaloids
- Narcotics/opioids
- Nonsteroidal anti-inflammatory drugs (NSAIDs)
- Triptans
- Miscellaneous other medications

Analgesics

- *Tylenol (acetaminophen)*: No adverse signs or symptoms in infant or negative effect on lactation; AAP considers it compatible with breastfeeding. Hales Lactation Risk Category 1 (safest category).

- *Aspirin (salicylate)*: Associated with Reye syndrome in infants; AAP guidelines are to use with caution; Hale Lactation Risk Category 3.
- *Excedrin (acetaminophen-aspirin-caffeine combination)*: See comments for each individual component. Caffeine can cause irritability and poor sleeping pattern in infants. Hales Lactation Risk Category 1 for acetaminophen, Category 3 for aspirin, and Category 2 for caffeine.

> **Box 8-2**
>
> My preferred analgesic for women who are breastfeeding is acetaminophen [Tylenol (acetaminophen)].

I prefer that my pregnant patients use Tylenol (acetaminophen) instead of Excedrin (acetaminophen-aspirin-caffeine), but if a woman feels Excedrin works better for her headaches, I caution her to limit its use to no more than twice a week to prevent rebound headache and to minimize irritability in her infant.

Antiemetics (Antinausea Medications)

- *Reglan (metoclopramide)*: No adverse events reported in infants; may aggravate depression in women and has recently been linked to a rare risk of tardive dyskinesia. Reglan is often used in infants for reflux (gastrointestinal) conditions. Hales Lactation Risk Category 2.
- *Zofran (ondansetron)*: No data available in infants. Hales Lactation Risk Category 2. Conveniently comes in an orally dissolving tablet (ODT), as well as in a regular tablet.
- *Compazine (prochlorperazine)*: Caution suggested; increased risk of apnea in this class of medication, called the phenothiazines.

Increased prolactin level can occur. Hales Lactation Risk Category 3.

- *Phenergan (promethazine)*: Sedation and apnea can occur in younger infants; do not use if infant is at high risk for apnea. Has been used for many years in pediatric patients for vomiting. Hales Lactation Risk Category 2.
- *Tigan (trimethobenzamide)*: Rarely used in infants; Hales Lactation Risk Category 4.

BOX 8-3

My preferred antinausea medications for women who are breastfeeding are Reglan (metoclopramide), Zofran (ondansetron), and Phenergan (promethazine). These can often help the headache in addition to the nausea.

Ergots and Ergot Alkaloids

This class of migraine medication includes treatments such as Cafergot (ergotamine-caffeine), Ergostat (ergotamine), and dihydroergotamine (DHE) in nasal spray and injectable formulations. Ergotamine can cause vomiting, diarrhea, and convulsions in doses used in migraine medications; it can also decrease milk production. There is some evidence that DHE is safer than ergotamine but for now the AAP instructs use with caution. Hales Lactation Risk Category 4.

BOX 8-4

I recommend that women avoid the ergot/ergotamine class of acute migraine medications while breastfeeding.

Narcotics/Opioids

This class of medication is considered addictive and often highly sedative. However, these drugs may be needed on occasion if a migraine has become severe and is not responsive to other treatment. Sedation in the infant as well as the mother can be a side effect. I recommend only using this class of medication if necessary to rescue a severe migraine attack. If used too often, it can lead to rebound and daily headache.

- *Stadol nasal spray (butorphanol)*: The AAP considers it compatible with breastfeeding. Could possibly cause sedation in the infant. Hales Lactation Risk Category 2.
- *Codeine*: The AAP considers it compatible with breastfeeding. Several rare cases of infant apnea have been associated with high doses. Hales Lactation Risk Category 3.
- *Vicodin (hydrocodone)*: Can cause infant drowsiness, apnea, or constipation. Hales Lactation Risk Category 3.
- *Demerol (meperidine)*: The AAP considers it compatible with breastfeeding. Can cause sedation, poor suckling reflex (poor feeding), and neurobehavioral delays in the infant. Hales Lactation Risk Category 2, but 3 if used just after delivery in early postpartum period.
- *Oxycodone*: Can cause sedation and gastrointestinal effects in infants. Hales Lactation Category 3.

Box 8-5

I recommend that women avoid the opioid class of medications. If your physician feels it absolutely necessary, he or she should prescribe codeine or butorphanol sparingly.

Nonsteroidal Anti-Inflammatory Drugs

This class of medication can be very useful in the treatment of headache for breastfeeding women, who often report their migraines are mild enough to treat with an anti-inflammatory like Motrin (ibuprofen) or Naproxen (Naprosyn) without the need for a triptan or pain medication. This is especially true during the early months of breastfeeding when the ovaries are still fairly "quiet" and ovulation has often not yet returned. For the most part, NSAIDs are quite safe during breastfeeding.

- *Voltaren, Cambia (diclofenac)*: No published evidence. Hales Lactation Risk Category 2.
- *Motrin, Advil (ibuprofen)*: No adverse signs or symptoms in infant or any negative effect on lactation. The AAP considers it compatible with breastfeeding. Often used for high fever in infants. Hales Lactation Risk Category 1.
- *Indomethacin*: One seizure reported in a 7-day-old infant. The AAP considers it compatible with breastfeeding. Hales Lactation Risk Category 3.
- *Toradol (ketorolac)*: No adverse effects on infants in one study. The AAP considers it compatible with breastfeeding. Hales Lactation Risk Category 2.
- *Aleve, Anaprox (naproxen, Naprosyn)*: One reported case of prolonged bleeding, hemorrhage, and anemia in a 7-day-old infant. The AAP considers it compatible with breastfeeding. Hales Lactation Risk Category 3.

Box 8-6

Of the available NSAIDs, Motrin (ibuprofen) is preferred. The others are considered generally okay.

Triptans

This class of migraine medication has become the standard of care for the acute treatment of migraine attacks in most adults. Most women will be on triptans before pregnancy, and, like Lisa, will want to know if they can resume their triptan during breastfeeding. Fortunately,

Imitrex (sumatriptan) is considered compatible with breastfeeding by the AAP. The other triptans are not listed in the AAP table, yet are not considered dangerous for breastfeeding; rather, there is simply not yet enough evidence to rate them. The common practice has been to pump and discard the breast milk for 6–8 hours after using any triptan other than sumatriptan. To minimize the amount of triptan that gets into the breast milk, women are often encouraged to take their triptan right after breastfeeding.

- *Axert (almotriptan)*: No published evidence. Hales Lactation Risk Category 3.
- *Relpax (eletriptan)*: Limited information shows that maternal doses up to 80 mg a day (the maximum daily dose) result in low levels of the drug in breast milk and no adverse effects in the infant, especially if the infant is less than 2 months old. Hales Lactation Risk Category 2.
- *Frova (frovatriptan)*: No published evidence. Long half-life of 25–30 hours; short-acting alternative may be preferred. Hales Lactation Risk Category 3.
- *Amerge (naratriptan)*: No published evidence. Next longest half-life to frovatriptan; shorter-acting triptans preferred. Hales Lactation Risk Category 3.
- *Maxalt (rizatriptan)*: No published evidence. Hales Lactation Risk Category 3.
- *Imitrex (sumatriptan)*: The AAP considers it compatible with breastfeeding. Hales Lactation Risk Category 3.
- *Zomig (zolmitriptan)*: No published evidence. Hales Lactation Risk Category 3.

My first choice is Imitrex (sumatriptan). My second choice is Relpax (eletriptan).

Miscellaneous

- *Fiorinal, Fioricet, Esgic (butalbital)*: Not recommended. Sedation in infant is a concern. Hales Lactation Category 3.

- *Caffeine*: Usual dietary amounts of caffeine are compatible with breastfeeding. Higher doses in combination products with aspirin and acetaminophen are not recommended owing to irritability and poor sleeping effects on the infant. Hales Lactation Risk Category 2 for Caffeine.
- *Isometheptene*: One of ingredients in Midrin; no published evidence. Potential risk of infant stimulation. Hales Lactation Risk Category 3.
- *Lidocaine*: The AAP considers it compatible with breastfeeding. Hales Lactation Risk Category 2.
- *Magnesium*: The AAP considers it compatible with breastfeeding. Hales Lactation Risk Category 1.
- *Prednisone (steroids)*: The AAP considers it compatible with breastfeeding. Degree and amount of exposure should be limited; prolonged exposure could result in growth and development issues for the infant. Inhaled or intranasal steroids may be preferable to oral steroids to limit infant exposure. Hales Lactation Risk Category 2.
- *Ultram (tramadol)*: No published evidence. Sedation in infant is a concern, although it hasn't been officially reported in studies. Hales Lactation Risk Category 2.

Preventive Medications and Breastfeeding

Most preventive medications that a woman takes before pregnancy can be resumed during breastfeeding if a daily preventive is needed. Preventives can be divided into three main categories: antihypertensives (blood pressure medications), antiepileptics (AEDs), and antidepressants.

Antihypertensives and Safety in Breastfeeding

Antihypertensives include beta-blockers, calcium-channel blockers, and a third category comprising miscellaneous others. Beta-blockers are most commonly used for migraine prevention; two of them are FDA approved for migraine prevention: Inderal (propanolol) and timolol.

Beta-Blockers

- *Inderal (propanolol):* The AAP considers it compatible with breastfeeding. Hales Lactation Risk Category 2.
- *Timolol:* The AAP considers it compatible with breastfeeding. Hales Lactation Risk Category 2.
- *Atenolol:* Cyanosis and low heart rate in the infant has been reported. The AAP urges caution if given to infants. Secretion into breast milk is much higher than for propanolol. Hales Lactation Risk Category 3.
- *Metoprolol:* The AAP considers it compatible with breastfeeding. Hales Lactation Risk Category 3.
- *Labetalol:* The AAP considers it compatible with breastfeeding. Hales Lactation Risk Category 2.

Inderal (propanolol), timolol, and labetalol are preferred over atenolol and metoprolol.

Calcium-Channel Blockers

- *Verapamil:* The AAP considers it compatible with breastfeeding. Hales Lactation Risk Category 2.

Other Blood Pressure Medications

- *Zestril (lisinopril):* The effects of Zestril on infants are unknown. Hales Lactation Risk Category 3.
- *Atacand (candesartan):* The effects on infants are unknown. Hales Lactation Risk Category 3.
- *Hydrochlorothiazide:* A diuretic; no complications have been reported in infant, but may reduce milk supply. Hales Lactation Risk Category 2.

Antiepileptics and Safety in Breastfeeding

- *Topamax (topiramate)*: No pediatric adverse effects have been found. Hales Lactation Risk Category 3.
- *Depakote (valproic acid)*: The AAP considers it compatible with breastfeeding. Hales Lactation Risk Category 2.
- *Zonegran (zonisamide)*: No complications have been found in infants, yet levels in the infant have been reported as high. It is not recommended during breastfeeding. Hales Lactation Risk Category 5.
- *Neurontin (gabapentin)*: No complications have been found in infants. Hales Lactation Risk Category 2.

Antidepressants and Safety in Breastfeeding

- *Elavil (amitriptyline)*: Across several studies, no adverse effects on infants were found. Hales Lactation Risk Category 2.
- *Pamelor (nortriptyline)*: Across several studies, no adverse effects on infants were found. Hales Lactation Risk Category 2.
- *Prozac (fluoxetine)*: According to the AAP, may cause colic, irritability, feeding, sleep disturbances, and slow weight gain in infants. Use in older infants (4–6 months or older) is safe since they can metabolize the medication more rapidly. Hales Lactation Risk Category 2.
- *Zoloft (sertraline)*: Transfer of the medication to the infant is minimal in several studies; no adverse effects on infants have been seen. Hales Lactation Risk Category 2.
- *Paxil (paroxetine)*: No adverse effects on infants in several studies. Hales Lactation Risk Category 2.
- *Celexa (citalopram)*: Two cases of excessive sleepiness, decreased feeding, and weight loss have been reported. Hales Lactation Risk Category 2.
- *Lexapro (escitalopram)*: No adverse effects in infants have been reported; the infant dose is less than an equivalent amount of

Celexa (citalopram) so Lexapro would be preferred over Celexa. Hales Lactation Risk Category 2.

- *Effexor (venlafaxine)*: No complications have been reported during breastfeeding. Hales Lactation Risk Category 3.
- *Wellbutrin (bupropion)*: One case of seizure in a 6-month-old was reported, and it may suppress milk production. Hales Lactation Risk Category 3.

Other Preventive Medications and Safety in Breastfeeding

- *Prednisone*: A steroid; the AAP considers prednisone compatible with breastfeeding. There is no adverse effect on the infant if used short-term. Therefore, a short course of prednisone to break a prolonged migraine would be safe, but long-term use with daily dosing during breastfeeding is not recommended. Hales Lactation Risk Category 2.
- *Magnesium sulfate*: The AAP considers it compatible with breastfeeding. Hales Lactation Risk Category 1.
- *Vitamin B$_2$ (riboflavin)*: The AAP considers it compatible with breastfeeding. Hales Lactation Risk Category 1.
- *Estrogen/progesterone contraceptive pill*: In rare cases, may cause breast enlargement and/or decrease in milk production and protein content. The AAP considers it compatible with breastfeeding. A better choice is progesterone in pill form such as Micronor and Nor-QD.

All the nonpharmacologic treatments discussed for migraine prevention during pregnancy would be appropriate during breastfeeding as well.

As the infant grows and breastfeeding decreases, the risk of medication effects to the child is expected to decrease due to several factors, including the infant's improved ability to metabolize and eliminate the medication. Also, as other foods and liquids are introduced, breast milk becomes only a part of the infant's diet and, therefore, the medication level plays a smaller role in the overall diet.

References

1. Rasmussen BK. Migraine and tension-type headache in a general population: precipitating factors, female hormones, sleep pattern and relation to lifestyle. Pain. 1993; 53: 65–72.

2. MacGregor EA. Migraine in pregnancy and lactation: a clinical review. J Fam Plan Reprod Health Care. 2007; 33(2): 83–93.

3. Marcus DA, Scharff L, Turk D. Longitudinal prospective study of headache during pregnancy and postpartum. Headache. 1999; 39: 625–632.

4. Evans RW, Loder EW. Migraine with aura during pregnancy. Headache. 2001: 43: 80–84.

5. Melhado EM, Maciel JA Jr, Guerreiro CA. Headache during gestation: evaluation of 1101 women. Can J Neurol Sci. 2007; 34: 187–192.

6. Cupini LM, Matteis M, Troisi E, et al. Sex-hormone-related events in migrainous females. A clinical comparative study between migraine with aura and migraine without aura. Cephalalgia. 1995; 15: 140–144.

7. Koren G, Pastuszak A, Ito S. Drugs in pregnancy. N Engl J Med. 1998; 338: 1128–1137.

8. Lucas S. Medication use in the treatment of migraine during pregnancy and lactation. Curr Pain Headache Rep. 2009; 13: 392–398.

9. Adeney KL, Williams MA, Miller RS, et al. Risk of preeclampsia in relation to maternal history of migraine headaches. J Matern Fetal Neonatal Med. 2005; 18: 167–172.

10. Li DK, Liu L, Odouli R. Exposure to non-steroidal anti-inflammatory drugs during pregnancy and risk of miscarriage: population based cohort study. Br Med J. 2003; 327: 368.

11. Sumatriptan Pregnancy Registry Interim Report January 1, 1996 through October 31, 2010.

12. Nezvalova-Henrikson K, Spigset O, Nordeng H. Triptan exposure during pregnancy and the risk of major congenital malformation

and adverse pregnancy outcomes: results from the Norwegian Mother and Child Cohort Study. Headache. 2010; 50: 563–575.

13. Kallen B, Lygner PE. Delivery outcome in women who used drugs for migraine during pregnancy with special reference to suma-triptan. Headache. 2001; 41: 351–356.

14. Holroyd KA, O'Donnell FJ, Stensland M, et al. Management of chronic tension-type headache with tricyclic antidepressant medication, stress management therapy, and their combination: a randomized controlled trial. JAMA. 2001; 285: 2208–2215.

15. Scharff L, Marcus DA, Turk DC. Maintenance of effects in the nonmedical treatment of headaches during pregnancy. Headache. 1996; 36: 285–290.

16. American Academy of Pediatrics Committee on Drugs. The trans-fer of drugs and other chemicals into human milk. Pediatrics. 2001; 108: 776–789.

17. Hale T. *Medications and Mothers' Milk* 2008. 13th ed. Amarillo, TX: Hale Publishing, LP.

18. National Library of Medicine LactMed Database. 2006. Toxnet. nlm.nih.gov/cgi-bin/sis/htmlgen?LACT Accessed October 1, 2010.

9

Women Helping Women

L ET'S REVISIT THE LIVES OF BETH, LISA, NANCY, Melanie, Theresa, Christine, and Kate. Each of these women has a unique story to tell about her migraine history and treatment. My hope is that you can find parts of your own story in those of one or more of these women. Their stories may become "your story" as you gain inspiration and information to successfully treat your migraines.

BETH

Beth is 19 years old, in college, and pre-med. She initially went to her gynecologist's office for birth control and was put on a low-dose birth control pill called Yasmin. After several months, her menstrual migraines started to get worse. When she called her gynecologist's office, a nurse instructed her to stop the pill in view of her worsening headaches. However, the nurse failed to ask her where in the pill pack the migraines were worse. The reality is that the migraines were worse when she was on the fourth week in the pill pack and on the placebo pills. It is likely that the lack of estrogen was the trigger for her menstrual migraines worsening, not the estrogen-containing "active" pills in the pack.

Beth was frustrated and went back to the gynecologist's office wondering if there was a different birth control pill that would be better for her. She needed birth control. Additionally, she wanted predictable, light periods and relief from her premenstrual syndrome (PMS) and premenstrual dysphoric disorder (PMDD) symptoms. The nurse practitioner she saw suggested Yaz instead of Yasmin. She explained to Beth that Yaz has 24 active pills and only 4 days of placebo; it is a "24/4" pill pack instead of the "21/7" of Yasmin. In addition, Yaz is approved by the U.S. Food and Drug Administration (FDA) for PMDD.

Several months later, Beth returns to the nurse practitioner. Her menstrual migraines are limited to the 4 days that she is on the placebo pills at the end of the Yaz. During that time, she takes Imitrex (sumatriptan) 100 mg up to twice a day for 4 days. Her PMDD symptoms are better, but she still finds herself irritable and on edge for the 5 days leading up to her period. The nurse practitioner prescribes Zoloft (sertraline) at 50 mg a day and tells her it is okay to increase the dose to 75–100 mg around her period if the 50 mg is not enough.

At the encouragement of a family friend, Beth came to see me. She asked, "What else can I do for my menstrual migraines? They come predictably when I am on my period and on the placebo pills. I'm concerned since I find myself taking eight Imitrex for these 4 days. I am not 100% better after the first dose, so I end up taking a second tablet each day for those 4 days. Also, I feel foggy and not 100% after taking the Imitrex. It's difficult for me to study and focus during this 4-day period each month. What would you recommend?"

My plan for Beth:

- Take the Yaz continuously for up to 3 months in a row; only cycle off and take the placebo every 3 months.
- Cycle off for only 4 days (this limits the drop in estrogen to 4 days instead of the traditional 7 days).
- When cycling off, wear a Vivelle (estradiol) dot 0.1 mg patch. This will prevent the drop in estrogen that is the main trigger for menstrual migraine.

- Take magnesium and vitamin B2 for migraine prevention; the total daily dose for each would be approximately 400 mg. Another option would be the combination product called Migrelief, which contains feverfew as well as B2 and magnesium in the recommended dosages for migraine prevention.
- Switch from Imitrex (sumatriptan) to Treximet. Treximet contains 500 mg of naproxen (a nonsteroidal anti-inflammatory drug or NSAID) combined with sumatriptan, and it may work better for Beth, producing less need to take a second tablet as she is currently doing. Also, from my experience, patients often report feeling more clear-headed after taking Treximet. Being clear-headed and returning to full function is very important for someone like Beth, who needs to focus on studying and getting good grades.
- Have Beth keep track of her migraines and any bleeding for 3 months and return back for a follow-up visit. She can go to www.headaches.org to print a headache calendar. She was instructed to bring her calendar with her on her follow-up visit.
- It's okay for Beth to continue on the Zoloft for her PMDD.
- Exercise, good nutrition, good sleep habits, and stress reduction management were also suggested to Beth as being part of an overall migraine treatment program.

Beth came to see me 3 months later. She reported mild break-through bleeding for a few days as she got used to taking the Yaz continuously. She liked not having a period or menstrual migraine every month. She cycled off for the week before she came in for her follow-up visit and tried the Treximet; she felt it worked faster and better than Imitrex. She was also relieved it did not upset her stomach despite the fact that it contains naproxen.

Beth's personal life had also changed. Ryan, her boyfriend, was upset with all the time she spent studying. He came over one evening to her dorm room, held up her books, and said "You have to pick. Is it me or the books?" She replied, "The books." He left upset and frustrated. I asked her how she was holding up. She had a great attitude "If he can't understand how important my studying is to me," she said,

> *"then he is not the kind of man for me!" I predict success for Beth, both personally and professionally. I was gratified to be able to play a part in lessening the burden of menstrual migraine for her as she moves forward. I will plan to see her every 3–6 months while referring her back to her gynecologist's office with a copy of her evaluation. A good headache specialist should openly communicate with other treating providers and let them do as much of the follow-up as they feel comfortable.*

❖

LISA

Lisa is the 25-year-old school teacher with disabling migraines, including menstrual migraines, and endometriosis. Her husband, Rick, was unsympathetic to her and does not understand why she can't just "suck it up" and deal with having a headache. She was taking Excedrin (acetaminophen-aspirin-caffeine combination) for her mild to moderate migraines, saving her Imitrex (sumatriptan) for her more severe migraines. She was told by her obstetrician-gynecologist that pregnancy could help both her migraines and endometriosis. She had also read that the ideal time to get pregnant is when a woman is 25–29 years old.

When Lisa came in to see me, she was on a continuous low-dose birth control pill, Loestrin 1/30, to prevent the endometriosis from returning. Despite taking Loestrin, she was getting pelvic pain and cramps. One year ago, she had laparoscopy and laser treatment for her endometriosis, which was diagnosed as moderate to severe by her gynecologist. She has a lot of questions about how to treat her menstrual and nonmenstrual migraines when she goes off the pill and begins trying to get pregnant. She also needs guidance on tapering off her daily preventive, Zonegran (zonisamide). Lisa's obstetrician-gynecologist tells her to make sure she is taking 0.4 mg folic acid daily, even before she goes off the birth control pill, to help prevent her baby from having a neural tube defect.

Lisa also suffers from generalized anxiety disorder (GAD). She worries a lot, has trouble relaxing, and has tight muscles in her neck. Now, worrying about getting pregnant, she lies awake at night.

My plan for Lisa:

- Take the folic acid 0.4 mg as recommended by her gynecologist's office.
- Taper off the daily preventive.
- Focus on nonpharmacologic treatment for the anxiety and migraines in view of upcoming pregnancy. Such treatment can include biofeedback, relaxation exercises, stress reduction, and cognitive-behavioral therapy (CBT). The CBT can help change Lisa's negative thinking and worry into a more positive attitude toward everything in her life. Most likely, I would refer Lisa to a licensed psychologist or therapist to help with this treatment plan.
- Marriage counseling is recommended. Both Lisa and Rick feel resentment toward each other. Rick is very healthy, headache-free, and does not understand Lisa's complaints and tears when she is suffering from a migraine. Lisa resents what she perceives as Rick's unwillingness to see migraine as a legitimate medical condition. She wants him to know that she wishes she didn't suffer with migraines and that she would much prefer to be headache-free and fully functional at all times.
- A regular exercise program, good eating habits, and improved sleep are encouraged.
- Excedrin and Imitrex are okay to continue, in my opinion, while Lisa is trying to get pregnant, but this should be reevaluated once she becomes pregnant. Both Excedrin and Imitrex should be limited to a maximum of twice a week to prevent rebound headache.
- Lisa should try Tylenol (acetaminophen) for her milder headaches instead of Excedrin since Tylenol is safe to take during pregnancy, but Excedrin is best to avoid. Also, it is okay to drink a small amount of caffeine with the Tylenol and see if this combination can be a substitute for the Excedrin in view of the upcoming pregnancy.
- Lisa should keep track of her headaches with a calendar and bring the calendar in for a follow-up visit in 2–3 months.

- *She should notify me as soon as she knows she is pregnant. I can then work with her obstetrician in treating Lisa's migraines during pregnancy.*

Lisa went off the birth control pill and the Zonegran and got pregnant within 3 months. She had only mild headaches during her pregnancy and was able to control them with Tylenol. She saw me several weeks before delivery and asked about migraine treatment with breastfeeding. I reassured her that she could resume her Imitrex for migraines during the postpartum period. As discussed in Chapter 8, the American Academy of Pediatrics lists Imitrex as compatible with breastfeeding; there is no need to pump and discard breast milk after taking Imitrex. I cautioned her on taking Excedrin as the caffeine in the Excedrin could cause some irritability and jitteriness in her infant; however, in moderation it would probably be okay. Still, a better medication for mild-moderate migraine during breastfeeding, in my opinion, would be ibuprofen (Advil or Motrin) or naproxen (Aleve).

Lisa delivered a healthy 7-pound baby boy and named him Tyler. She had only mild headaches in the first 3 months of breastfeeding and only needed Aleve to get through them. After 3 months, her migraines returned and she resumed taking Imitrex for them. She felt better knowing that the Imitrex would not hurt her baby. She is now job-sharing with another teacher and enjoying raising her son. She and her husband, Rick, are working on their issues in marriage counseling and are considering trying to have another child in a year.

❖

NANCY

Nancy is the 29-year-old attorney with menstrual migraine, irritable bowel syndrome (IBS), posttraumatic stress disorder (PTSD), and a history of childhood abuse. In Chapter 7 we learned that she was taking as many as 6–12 Excedrin (acetaminophen-aspirin-caffeine) a day and had progressed from episodic migraine to an almost daily low-grade headache. She is now suffering from rebound headache and has "medication overuse" headache from her daily Excedrin use. She was referred to me by her primary care provider, who needed help getting her out of rebound.

My plan for Nancy:

- First, I wanted to educate her to the fact that her daily Excedrin use is the cause of her almost daily headache. Unless she is willing to stop the Excedrin (or limit its use), she will never get better. I explained to her that it may be hard for a few weeks but that her health is well worth it. I reassured her that I won't leave her without treatment to help prevent withdrawal headache as she gets off the Excedrin. She could either stop the Excedrin abruptly or slowly go off it. I offered her a "bridge" of treatment to help her during this withdrawal period in the form of a long-acting triptan such as Frova (frovatriptan) with naproxen twice a day for 7–10 days, and a steroid (prednisone) for break-through headache.

- I suggested we begin a plan to prevent her migraines and help her other medical conditions. I recommended Zoloft (sertraline) for her PTSD and IBS and Topamax (topiramate) for migraine prevention. Nancy was instructed to start only one new daily medication at a time so it would be easy to track side effects and where they were coming from. Both will be started at a low dose and increased gradually.

- Nancy should address the PTSD and abuse issue with her therapist.

- Nancy is encouraged to try relaxation exercises, stress-reduction activities such as a regular exercise program, getting together with girlfriends, and generally making a life for herself outside of work.

- I offered to fill out a Family Medical Leave Act (FMLA) form for her to have on file at her workplace (available if a company has 50 or more employees). This will protect her from losing her job from missed absences due to migraine attacks.

- *Acute migraine medication should be limited to a maximum of two doses a week to prevent rebound. Acute medication could be a triptan such as Imitrex (sumatriptan) or a combined triptan/NSAID medication, such as Treximet.*
- *Good health habits were encouraged, including attention to a healthy diet and adequate sleep.*
- *Nancy should come back to the doctor's office in 2–4 weeks and check in by phone every 3–4 days with a progress report to help her during withdrawal from the Excedrin.*

On a follow-up visit several months later, Nancy reported improvement in her migraines, IBS symptoms, and stress level. She was taking Topamax at 100 mg and Zoloft at 100 mg after gradually increasing the dose of both. With the help of her therapist, she realized that her workplace was too stressful for her. She accepted a job working as in-house counsel for a company and left the big law firm. She had better work hours and felt much less stressed when she left her office at the end of the day. Going to the gym after work became part of her daily routine. She is still seeing Keith, an attorney, but has recently met Steve, a 32-year-old pharmaceutical rep, at her gym. She is attracted to Steve's enthusiasm and optimistic outlook on life. His optimism is rubbing off on her. Life is good! She still gets a migraine once or twice a month but the attack is easily treated if she takes a Treximet (sumatriptan/naproxen) early in the attack. She no longer takes daily Excedrin.

❖

MELANIE

Melanie is the 35-year-old mother of two young children. She came in suffering from severe menstrual migraines lasting up to 7 days straight. In addition, she suffers from major depression. She was also recently diagnosed with fibromyalgia and put on Elavil (amitriptyline). She started with 10 mg of Elavil at night and was told to increase by 10 mg every week until she got up to 50 mg. However, when I saw her, she was taking 30 mg, becoming constipated, and had dry mouth and fatigue. The Elavil had lessened the tightness in her neck muscles but was not helping her depression. She had read that Elavil might cause weight gain, which depressed her further since she was already 15–20 pounds overweight. She came to see me since she read on my website that I specialize in mood disorders as well as headache.

When I asked Melanie what brought her to my office, she began to cry: "Everything!" she replied. "My migraines are horrible, especially around my period; my muscles hurt all over my body; I am depressed; and was recently told I have fibromyalgia! This can't be happening to me. I have two small children who need me. My husband travels a lot, and I often feel like a single parent. Recently I have been yelling at my kids and then afterward I feel guilty."

- *Melanie was already on the following medications:*
- *Maxalt (rizatriptan) at 10 mg as needed for migraine*
- *Elavil at 30 mg nightly for fibromyalgia and migraine prevention*
- *Soma (carisoprodol; a muscle relaxant) at 350 mg as needed for tight muscles*
- *Vicodin (hydrocodone) at 7.5 mg as needed for severe migraine when the Maxalt is not enough*

My plan for Melanie:

- *Take Cymbalta (duloxetine) at 30 mg every morning for 2 weeks with breakfast; then, if tolerated well after 2 weeks, increase to 60 mg every morning. The Cymbalta is to treat her depression and fibromyalgia. Cymbalta is FDA approved to treat both major depressive disorder and fibromyalgia. Unlike Elavil, Cymbalta causes no weight gain in clinical trials with women. There was also no sexual dysfunction reported. Finally, Cymbalta may help with migraine prevention, although it is not FDA-approved for this condition. So I am hoping Cymbalta can help with all three of Melanie's medical conditions: the depression, fibromyalgia, and migraines.*

- *Take the Patient Health Questionnaire (PHQ-9) screening for depression to give me a baseline for Melanie's degree of depression. From there we would be able to monitor her progress with future screenings. The PHQ-9 is available on the Internet.*
- *Taper off the Elavil in view of its side effects (constipation, weight-gain, dry month, and fatigue).*
- *For her menstrual migraine, begin naproxen sodium at 550 mg twice a day several days before her anticipated menstrual migraine. Continue until the end of her period. This short-term prevention of menstrual migraine with a nonsteroidal anti-inflammatory can be effective and inexpensive.*
- *Maxalt at 10 mg for her migraines. It can be repeated after 2 hours for a maximum of 30 mg or three tablets in 24 hours. She can take the naproxen or Motrin at the same time as the Maxalt when her migraine is occurring.*
- *Stop the Soma and Vicodin, which are both addictive and can cause sleepiness. The Vicodin can cause medication overuse and rebound headache.*
- *Develop an exercise program, which has been found to help fibromyalgia.*
- *Begin physical therapy and/or massage therapy to help with her tight muscles and fibromyalgia pain.*
- *Start seeing to a licensed therapist and/or psychologist for relaxation training, biofeedback, and CBT.*
- *Take 1 tablet of Migrelief (magnesium, B-2, feverfew) twice a day and Petadolex (butterbur) at 75 mg twice a day. These are herbal preventives that can work with the Cymbalta as part of Melanie's overall migraine prevention program.*

Melanie returned 3 months later. Her fibromyalgia and depression were better. She really likes both the physical therapist and the marriage and family therapist that she has been seeing. She has started taking an exercise class at the local gym and was getting more involved with her children's school. However, she needs a lot of Maxalt for her menstrual migraines. She only gets nine tablets a month and takes two tablets a day, on the average, for up to 5–7 days in a row. She requests a prescription for Vicodin or Fioricet (butalbital) for those days when she has a migraine and has no more Maxalt left. She argues that none of the over the counter medications is strong enough for her menstrual migraines. I replace Maxalt with Frova (frovatriptan) since both are triptan medications, but Frova lasts longer than Maxalt and can be especially useful for prolonged migraines (its effects can last up to 26 hours). Melanie can still take Motrin or Aleve with the Frova. I recommend the following:

- Take Frova 2.5 mg with two tablets of Aleve at the first sign of menstrual migraine.
- Repeat the Frova if necessary after 2 hours; maximum daily dose is 7.5 mg or three tablets in 24 hours. Ideally, however, she would only need one tablet of Frova a day.
- Consider taking the Frova as an "off-label" short-term preventive treatment.

Frova is not FDA approved to be taken for prevention of menstrual migraine. However, I have often used this approach for patients like Melanie who suffer from a predictable 5- to 7-day menstrual migraine. Just because a medication is not FDA approved for a particular situation does not mean we can't go "off- label" to help a patient's suffering. However, as healthcare providers, we do have a responsibility to make sure that what we are prescribing is safe. I feel that Frova can safely be used in a short-term preventive strategy for menstrual migraine, but always follow your own doctor's recommendations.

❖

THERESA

Theresa is the 40-year-old woman in the middle of a divorce. She is struggling with migraines, as well as insomnia and stress. She also has a lot of sinus symptoms and feels that nasal congestion and allergy symptoms may lead to some of her migraines. Her sinus and allergy symptoms are *worse in the fall and spring, and this is also when her migraines are more frequent. However, over-the-counter allergy medications and decongestants only give her partial relief. Migraine medications like Maxalt (rizatriptan) and Imitrex (sumatriptan) do not completely relieve her congestion but do help her headaches. Theresa's primary care provider gave her a prescription for Ambien (zolpidem) for insomnia; it helps Theresa get to sleep, but she is unable to stay asleep. Also, she fears becoming addicted to it. Feeling miserable and now averaging two or three headaches a week, Theresa's worst headaches are occurring around her period and are sometimes lasting for up to 4 days.*

My plan for Theresa:

- *See a licensed therapist or psychologist to work with her on the stress of her divorce and to address her insomnia and migraines.*
- *Begin stress-reduction measures, including regular exercise.*
- *Decide on a consistent time for going to bed and getting up at the same time every day; migraines can be triggered by not enough or too much sleep, as well as poor-quality sleep.*
- *Melatonin ER (extended release) for insomnia is recommended instead of Ambien. Melatonin is available over-the-counter and has been helped many headache patients get to sleep, stay asleep, and have fewer headaches. In my opinion, most migraine sufferers can safely take melatonin every evening without the risk of addictiveness. Other options would be Benadryl (diphenhydramine) or Periactin (cyproheptadine). Benadryl and Periactin are both sedating antihistamines and may help her allergies as well.*
- *Undergo a trial for 2 weeks with a steroid nasal spray like Flonase, Nasacort, or Nasonex. She can use two sprays each nostril once a day and see if she has less nasal congestion and possibly fewer headaches. This treatment approach has been useful in my practice for patients who suffer from both allergies and migraines.*
- *Start taking Petadolex (butterbur) and Migrelief (B$_2$, magnesium, and feverfew) for migraine prevention.*
- *Keep a headache diary and return back in 2 months.*

Theresa came back after 2 months with her headache diary. The nasal steroid spray had been helpful in reducing nasal congestion and allergy symptoms. Her migraines got better initially after beginning the Melatonin ER 3 mg and meeting with the therapist. However, the divorce was getting very stressful, and her husband has been threatening to "ruin her" financially. She suspected he was hiding some of his money. She has been feeling on edge and getting irritable with her sons and well-meaning friends. Recently, she snapped uncharacteristically at one of her best friends, telling her: "This is my divorce, not yours! Let me handle it my way."

She told me that she's tired of everyone telling her what to do. Lately, she has thought it would be nice if she could just go to sleep and never wake up. She wonders, "Where is all the joy in life? The day-to-day stress of life with paying bills, going through this divorce, doing laundry and dealing with my teenage sons is just not worth the occasional moments of joy. Sometimes death sounds welcome."

I asked Theresa if she had any suicide plans and said replied, "No, I would never actually hurt myself, especially since I have two sons who count on me. But just not waking up one morning would be fine with me."

I had Theresa fill out the PHQ-9 depression questionnaire, and her score showed moderate to severe depression. I discussed various antidepressants with her and we agreed on Cymbalta (duloxetine), with reassurance that Cymbalta does not cause weight gain or sexual dysfunction. I also told her there was a chance that Cymbalta could help preventing her headaches. She would still need a triptan like Maxalt (rizatriptan)or Imitrex (sumatriptan) for acute migraine treatment, but may find that her migraines are less frequent and less severe.

Theresa's treatment plan:

- Begin Cymbalta at 30 mg every morning with breakfast for 2 weeks and then increase to 60 mg.
- Address her negative thinking in counseling. CBT might help for her migraine and insomnia.

- *Consider Topamax (topiramate) if her migraines do not decrease in frequency with the Cymbalta.*
- *Come back for a follow-up visit in 1 month; check in by e-mail or phone call between now and then.*
- *Get Theresa's permission to discuss her case with her therapist. This "team" approach is critical for optimal care.*
- *Give Theresa the names and contact information for several local divorce recovery workshops. It is important for Theresa to not feel alone as she struggles with her divorce.*
- *Encourage her to stay connected with her support system of family and friends. Encourage distance with friends or family members who drain her emotionally or are unhealthy. She needs to surround herself with emotionally stable friends and family as she works through the divorce.*

Two years later, Theresa comes in for a follow-up with her migraines. She looks wonderful and is full of self-confidence. The divorce has been final for over a year now. She works full-time, her sons are doing well, and she is training to be a facilitator for the divorce recovery workshop that she attended 2 years ago. She is also considering going back to school to get her MBA. She still gets migraines with her period but takes her Maxalt at 10 mg and it works well. She has gone off the Cymbalta and is no longer depressed. She now looks back and thinks her "ex" did her a favor when he had an affair. She has not felt this happy in years. She has realized, through therapy, that her marriage had not been good for many years. She now feels "free" to move into all that life has to offer.

❖

CHRISTY

Christy is the 47-year-old with menstrual migraines and beginning perimenopause. I first met her 2 years ago when she had two emergency room visits in 1 week because of prolonged, disabling menstrual migraine. She did fine for over a year on Topamax (topiramate), but she was feeling miserable with hot flashes, night sweats, and irregular periods. She has had a tubal ligation and would prefer not to be on birth control pills; she had a bad experience in the past with going on a pill that caused weight gain and bloating. She had picked up an over-the-counter black cohosh supplement that is supposed to help hot flashes but it has not been very effective. She is also drinking soy milk and taking red clover. Her migraines are increasing. They used to occur only with her period but now they are occurring once or twice a week on average. She has been taking naproxen 550 mg and Imitrex (sumatriptan)100 mg, but when she came in, she was running out her nine tablets of Imitrex before the end of the month.

My plan for Christy:

- Wear Vivelle (estradiol) dot 0.025 mg and change it twice weekly to help alleviate the hot flashes, night sweats, and insomnia. Since the estrogen goes through the skin into the blood and bypasses the liver and stomach, Christy could find relief within 24 hours. It's best to start with the lowest dose necessary to help her symptoms.
- Cycle with progesterone if she begins to not have her period for 3 or more months. As long as she is still having periods, then I don't feel she needs progesterone.
- Consider Topamax (topiramate) since her migraines are occurring once or twice a week. Topamax can help prevent her migraines and lessen the severity of those she gets. Christy also finds the possible side effect of appetite suppression very appealing.
- Petadolex (butterbur) and Migrelief (B2, magnesium, and feverfew) are encouraged for migraine prevention.

Christy came back 2 months later thrilled with the results of the Vivelle dot and the Topamax. The estrogen has helped her hot flashes, night sweats, and insomnia. Her headaches are now milder, occurring less than once a week, and are more easily treated with Imitrex and naproxen. She heard that Botox (botulinum toxin) is now FDA approved for migraine prevention and wonders if she would be a candidate for *it, since it has recently been approved for chronic migraine (15 or more headache days a month). Unfortunately, unless Christy can document having 15 or more headache days a month, her insurance company won't cover it. I explained to Christy that I can still schedule her for a Botox injection visit but that she may have to pay out of pocket for it. She will consider this. In the meantime, she will continue her treatment regimen:*

- *Topamax: 100 mg at night*
- *Vivelle dot: 0.025 mg, applied and changed twice weekly*
- *Petadolex: 75 mg twice a day*
- *Migrelief: 1 tablet twice a day*
- *Imitrex: 100 mg with naproxen 550 mg for migraine attacks*
- *Naproxen: 550 mg alone for mild headache attacks*
- *Good health habits including diet, exercise, and sleep*

❖

KATE

Kate is in a good marriage. She and her husband Bob are the proud parents of three adult children. And yet, she has had disabling migraines for many years. They began when she was 15 years old and have always been associated with her periods. She has been completely menopausal, with no periods for a full year and has fewer migraine headaches. She is thrilled with fewer migraines but, like Christy, is struggling with hot flashes, night sweats, and insomnia. Her gynecologist gave her a prescription for hormones, but she has not filled it. She recently heard an alarming report on the nightly news about the increased risk of invasive breast cancer from a large study of women on hormones.

Kate came to my headache practice to get a second opinion. "Should I go on hormones like my gynecologist recommends?" she asks. "Is it safe? How will they affect my migraines?"

I told her that the decision of whether to go on hormones is an individual one. For most women in their early menopausal years, the benefits outweigh the risks. Women tend to be more symptomatic with hot flashes, night sweats, and insomnia during the first 3–5 years of menopause. To go on hormones at the beginning of menopause does not mean you'll be on them forever. The benefits and risks should be reevaluated with regular follow-up visits. Many women take a low-dose hormone product for 3–5 years and then stop.

Kate was worried that the hormone product would bring back her menstrual migraines—from which she was finally getting relief.

I told her that studies indicate that topical estrogen products, such as an estrogen patch or estrogen gel, are less likely to aggravate migraines in a woman with a history of migraines than are oral preparations. Also, bioidentical estrogen tends to be safer and often has fewer side effects than the synthetic estrogens.

Kate persists. She tells me that her friend Mary goes to a compounding pharmacy and gets an estrogen and progesterone capsule that is made up just for her. "Wouldn't that be better?" she asks.

There is no scientific evidence that compounded products are any safer than the commercially available products that have been FDA approved. In fact, compounded products are not subject to the same government-required testing and, therefore, could potentially be less safe. Here is what I recommend for Kate:

- *Vivelle (estradiol) dot 0.025 mg: Apply a patch and change twice weekly*
- *Prometrium (progesterone): 100 mg every evening*
- *Kate should monitor her headache pattern as hormone therapy is begun.*

Kate's dose of the Vivelle (estradiol) patch may need to be increased to give her enough relief from her menopausal symptoms. However, using the lowest dose necessary for the shortest amount of time necessary is consistent with current established guidelines for hormonal therapy. Kate is encouraged to go to www.menopause.org to learn more about the use of hormones, including bioidenticals, for menopausal symptoms.

> *On follow-up, Kate reports that she has gradually increased her Vivelle dot to her current 0.05 mg dose and changes her patch twice weekly. She continues to take Prometrium 100 mg every evening. Her migraines only occur about once or twice a month; her triggers include weather change and stress. She no longer suffers from menstrual migraines, and she is thrilled. However, she reports that she is very concerned about one of her employees, Claire. Claire is calling in sick 2–3 days a month because of "bad headaches," and these seem to take place about a month apart.*
>
> *Kate suspects Claire is suffering from monthly menstrual migraines. She asks if I am taking new patients in my practice.*

Kate is moving away from disabling migraines as she continues into her menopausal years. But for every Kate, there are many other women like Beth, Lisa, Nancy, Melanie, Theresa, Christy, and Claire, who continue to suffer from disabling menstrual migraines. Some of them have many years, even decades, before they experience menopause and possible relief. The good news is that there is hope and treatment available for these women. The specific treatment that works may be different for each woman but, importantly, treatment is available and can help. Never give up on finding effective treatment for your menstrual migraines. To give up on your headaches is to give up on yourself.

10

Headache and the Family

WHEN MY MOTHER WAS YOUNG, SHE REMEMBERS HER own mother going to bed for hours and days at a time because she did not feel well. My mother and her siblings were instructed to stay quiet and not bother their mother during these times. There was a housekeeper who took over much of the parenting when my grandmother felt ill. The housekeeper became more of a mother figure than their own mother for much of their growing-up years. Looking back, I suspect my grandmother had migraines.

"When I get a migraine, it's called 'pizza night' at my home. That's because my husband orders out pizza since I am too sick to cook dinner. That may sound like fun, but I am too sick to join my family for dinner. I am lying in the dark, in my bedroom, with my head throbbing."

❖

"My family and I were recently on vacation at a beautiful resort. Several days into our vacation, I began my period as well as a severe menstrual migraine. I was miserable in the hotel room, and we had to cut our vacation short. I just wanted to get home and be in my own bed."

❖

"When I get a migraine, every sound my children make bothers me. I have to tell them to turn the TV down, to speak softly, and take their shoes off. Even the sound of them walking around the house bothers me. I feel bad telling my kids they have to tip-toe around their own home but I have no choice."

❖

Do any of these scenarios sound familiar?

Migraine affects 1 out of every 4 households in the United States. It affects not just the migraine sufferer but everyone in the household. As these examples illustrate, the disability that a migraineur experiences carries over into the dynamics at home. Often, family members are asked to keep their voice down, turn the lights off, turn the TV down, get their own dinner, or do tasks that the migraine sufferer can no longer do because of the migraine attack. Not only is the woman with migraine in pain, but the whole family suffers as a result of her migraine attack.

It would seem natural that a nonmigraine family member would resent a family member's migraine attacks, given the disruption they cause within the family. Over time, the resentment of the migraine condition may transform into an overall resentment of the family member who suffers from the migraine headaches. In some cases, the family member may think that the headache sufferer is "making it up," just trying to get out of family responsibilities. I have often heard this comment: "It's just a headache. Get over it."

The reality is that migraine is not just a headache; it is disabling and can cause major disruption in someone's ability to function during a attack. Although it may seem unfair that other family members have to pick up the slack and take on more responsibility, this is the reality in most migraine households.

To illustrate, let's look at Melanie, the 35-year-old migraine sufferer who has two children, 5 and 7 years old. During a migraine attack, she is irritable and often yells at them. Sometimes, in reaction to the yelling, they start crying. She has had to miss activities at their school when in the middle of one of her bad menstrual migraine attacks. What will happen to her children and their attitude if this pattern continues?

They could begin to resent the disruption that their mother's migraines cause in their life. I have seen some children begin to mimic or copy their mother's complaints, complaining of headaches of their own. In some cases, the child may truly be suffering from migraine; in other cases, he or she may want attention, seeing "headache" as a way to stay home from school. I have seen cases in which the kids miss so much school they have to be home-schooled. Overall, a mother's disabling headaches can be very disruptive to creating a stable environment for children and teenagers. Spouses and significant others are often asked to take on more responsibility during migraine attacks. Over time, this extra burden can cause resentment and anger.

It is easy to sympathize with someone using crutches for a broken leg. Medical conditions with obvious evidence of disability are more easily accepted by those not afflicted. In the case of headache, there is usually no obvious external sign—the sufferer may look normal. Headache pain is considered "subjective" since it can't be measured objectively. Examples of objective pain could be the size of the cut or laceration, the severity of the broken bone, or the extent of the wound injury. But subjective pain refers to what the person is experiencing, and this is not measurable by others. It is one's own internal experience. This is a major source of frustration for migraine sufferers.

My advice for family members of migraine sufferers:

- Accept that migraine is a very real medical condition. In most cases, it is a chronic condition that produces episodic attacks.

Between attacks, the migraine patient may be able to fully function in all activities of daily life. In more severe cases, the individual may be so disabled she is not functioning well at all.

- Let your loved one know that you care and are sorry that she has to suffer during an attack. Let her know you want to be there for her and will do what you can to help her. However, it is okay to continue to live your life to its fullest, including going to family functions and activities that your spouse or significant other may not be able to attend. Your own life does not need to be "on hold" because of your loved one's migraines.

- Hold the sufferer accountable for practicing good health habits, including keeping to an exercise program, eating a healthy diet, getting enough sleep, and doing whatever she can to lessen the burden of migraine both in her own life and in the family unit.

- Consider coming along to some of the doctor appointments so you can understand the treatment plan, expectations, and possible side effects of the migraine treatments. In some cases, you may be of help by learning how to administer an injection for a severe migraine attack. This also shows that you are taking this condition seriously and want to help your loved one get better.

- Educate yourself about migraine. Several good websites include those offered by the National Headache Foundation (www.headaches.org), the American Headache Society Committee on Headache Education (www.achenet.org), and www.migraine.com.

- Be aware of triggers that can cause a migraine in your loved one, such as a skipped meal, travel, lack of sleep, or her period. You can encourage a proactive approach to control the known triggers and help your loved one get control of her migraines. However, accept the fact the migraine sufferer may be grumpy and irritable and not always appreciative of your well-meaning advice.

There are some things in life we can control; there are others we have no control over, like the family we were born into. (Research now suggests a genetic link to common migraine.) In most cases, migraine sufferers did nothing wrong to develop this condition. I reassure my patients of this fact constantly. However, there are supporting factors we can control, such as exercise, diet, sleep, caffeine and alcohol intake, and how we handle stress.

What To Do During a Migraine Attack

If your spouse is having a migraine attack and has effective medication to treat it, then I recommend you take the kids (if you have kids at home) and go out for a few hours. Most migraine attacks will get better faster if the sufferer can lie down and allow the medication to work. A quiet dark room can help since sensitivity to light and noise is often part of a migraine. If the kids are older and no longer at home, it can still be helpful for the spouse to leave for a few hours and allow the sufferer some peace and quiet. Going to the gym can be a great outlet. Being overly involved during an attack may be negatively received as being controlling. So, it may be wise to get out of the house.

After the Migraine Attack

Be aware that there is a period after the migraine attack in which the sufferer may still not feel 100%. During the hours after an attack, she may feel tired, unable to focus, or even feel a little spacey. As a result, don't expect her to jump right back into an accounting project or help the kids with homework. It may take another 24 hours for complete recovery. In the more complicated migraine cases, the person may not feel she ever returns to full function. In those cases in which the patient and family suspect that the migraine condition is complicated and keeping the patient from participating in family activities often, it would be worthwhile to seek out a headache evaluation at a specialized headache center or clinic like those listed on the websites previously mentioned (www.headaches.org and www.achenet.org).

Be Prepared for an Emergency Room Visit

In Chapter 11, I encourage migraine sufferers to keep a list of all prescription medications, allergies, and medical history. Here, I encourage family members to know where that list is and have a copy to take along to any unexpected emergency room or urgent care visit. This list can save valuable time and provide the medical staff with important medical information. Be aware of how the patient typically treats a migraine attack. Ideally, there is a rescue plan in place, such as an injectable medication that can be used at home to prevent an emergency room visit. In my headache practice, I do everything I can to make sure migraine patients have a rescue plan. However, there are times when a migraine attack is so severe that home rescue may not be possible.

Be prepared and know where to go to if a migraine attack is severe. An urgent care center can give injections for nausea and pain but, in most cases, cannot administer intravenous (IV fluids) or do a computed tomography (CT) scan of the brain. Therefore, if a migraine attack is severe and associated with vomiting or dehydration, it would be best to go to an emergency room where IV fluids can be given. Also, if the patient complains that "this is the worst headache" she has ever had, the emergency room is better than the urgent care, in case a brain scan is needed. In cases of head trauma, an emergency room is also better since the CT scan can look for a bleed in the brain, which can be a medical emergency and may need emergency surgery.

Have a plan in place for who can watch the kids while you are at the emergency room or urgent care setting. This could be a neighbor or family member. Have their phone numbers ready. This may all sound very basic, but it can be very helpful to be prepared. Having ready the list of medications, allergies, and medical history; knowing the location of the urgent care or emergency room; and having phone numbers of who to call to watch the kids can help lessen the stress of a severe migraine attack. A list of treating healthcare providers with their phone numbers can also be helpful. Depending on your insurance plan, you may need to call the primary care provider to "authorize" the emergency or urgent care visit, to make sure the visit will be covered by your insurance.

Always keep the headache provider aware of the situation and set up a follow-up appointment after any unexpected emergency room or urgent care visits. Often a change in medication or treatment is needed to prevent future emergency visits. Also, many patients are sent home from the emergency room with a narcotic or pain medication such as Vicodin (hydrocodone), and this is often not the ideal medication to continue. Many headache providers avoid narcotics because of their high addictive potential and the issue of rebound headache. Therefore, seeing the treating headache provider is an important follow-up after any emergency room or urgent care visit.

In addition, many headache specialists keep electronic records and can fax medical records to the emergency room or urgent care clinic to help the medical staff plan more effective treatment. In some cases, I fax the most recent headache visit directly to the patient to hand-carry to the emergency room or urgent care clinic. Find out whether your medical providers can fax or e-mail medical files to help with after-hours emergency care for headaches. In the case of my own practice, this system only works if I am called and told that my migraine patient is going in for emergency treatment. So, please call us (headache providers) if you or your loved one is going in for after-hours emergency treatment. Also, we may be able to call ahead and order a specific treatment; in some cases, we may have a "standing protocol" that we want the staff to use for treatment. We may have already prepared for you a printed protocol for after-hours treatment that can be handed to the staff upon your arrival. Having a written note or letter from your doctor can help legitimize the migraine condition and create less of a negative attitude on the part of the emergency staff. Keep in mind that some patients are considered "narcotic seeking" and come in to an emergency room complaining of a migraine and demanding Demerol (meperidine), Dilaudid (hydromorphone), or morphine: all powerful and addictive medications.

These narcotic-seeking migraine patients can cause the emergency staff to be suspicious of any migraine patient. But a written protocol from your specialist may include medications that are not addictive, such as antinausea medication, IV magnesium, Benadryl (diphenhydramine), steroids, and Toradol (ketorolac). Once the staff is aware that your loved one is not a narcotic-seeking migraine patient, their attitude often softens. One last note: Take a blanket to the emergency room, since waiting rooms often can be cold. Sunglasses can help with light sensitivity, and a plastic bag or basin can help if any nausea or vomiting occurs.

In recent months, I have been sending my patients to an infusion center instead of the emergency room. My patients can receive IV fluids and IV medications without the bright lights, noise, and chaos of the emergency room. However, most infusion centers are not open 24 hours a day and may require an appointment. This treatment approach works best when the diagnosis of migraine has been already made, and the treatment has already been fully discussed with the patient ahead of time.

Last, always request that copies of any emergency or urgent care visit be sent to your headache specialist. These copies provide valuable medical information for your treatment going forward.

My aim in this chapter was to equip the family members of migraine patients with the knowledge and tools needed to take care of their loved ones. But, more than anything, the desire and willingness to be educated and ready for any situation that comes is the best possible care. Keep up the good work. You and your loved ones will benefit. May you and your family enjoy life to the fullest despite the burden of migraine.

11

Finding Treatment and Resources for Migraine

IGRAINE SUFFERERS ARE OFTEN FRUSTRATED WITH healthcare providers who don't seem to understand how disabling their headaches are or don't have the time to listen to their headache history. To get the best care, you need to take charge of your treatment by choosing the right kind of specialist for your situation, preparing well, and bringing a complete treatment history to your appointment. Many physicians have appointments booked every 15 minutes, so it is crucial to get the most out of the limited time you have with your provider.

The Healthcare Team: Which Specialist to See?

A team approach involving all your treating providers is ideal; such an approach may be referred to as "multidisciplinary," in that the providers may represent different disciplines of medicine and healthcare. For example, our patient Lisa, who is considering pregnancy, has an obstetrician-gynecologist as well as a family medicine provider. She also sees a therapist for counseling. Other headache sufferers may also be seeing neurologists, psychiatrists, internists, pain specialists, chiropractors, acupuncturists, physical therapists, or psychologists. You are best served if all your treating providers are working as a team to help lessen the burden of migraine in your life.

Scheduling an Appointment with Your Primary Care Provider

If you like your current primary care provider, but feel that he or she doesn't have enough time to listen to you tell your headache story, then schedule a "headache-focused" visit. If you try to combine talking to your provider about your headaches at the same visit you are covering other medical issues, there may be not enough time to fully evaluate your headaches. That situation can be frustrating for you and your provider.

Scheduling this headache-focused visit will give you a good sense of how interested your primary care provider is in helping you with your migraine headaches. You may also be able to determine how up-to-date your doctor is with treatment options as he or she reviews your current treatment and offers recommendations and advice.

Preparing for Your Appointment

One of the most important ways to prepare for your appointment is to keep a headache diary or calendar of your headaches. I recommend that a diary be kept for at least 3 months before your appointment so a pattern can be seen. It also helps to mark down the first and last day of your period for each month to see if your migraines are related to your menstrual cycle.

Prepare a list of the medications you currently take for your headaches. If you are interested in trying something new, and have a particular medication in mind, tell your doctor.

Prepare another list of medications you have tried in the past that have either not worked for your migraines or that you have not been able to tolerate because of side effects or other issues.

I recommend you prepare and bring in a list of all your treating providers, with their contact information (office phone number, fax number, e-mail, mailing address); bring it to all your headache-related appointments. In some cases, you may be asked to sign a release form giving permission for providers to discuss your case. This type of communication can lead to better outcomes as your providers work as a team. In addition, this open communication can help eliminate repeat testing and provide for more efficient healthcare.

Bring your headache diary, menstruation diary, lists of medications, and contact information for your treating providers to your primary care appointment.

Making the Most of Your Appointment

First and foremost, be clear in your reasons for scheduling this headache-focused visit. Make sure your provider knows whether you want him or her to better manage your headaches or whether you are looking for a referral to a headache specialist.

During your appointment, give your physician a description of your headaches, focusing on the most recent 3–6 months. Are the headaches disabling? Is there any sensitivity to light or noise or smells? Is there nausea or vomiting? Has the diagnosis of migraine already been made? Tell your doctor how many headache days you are having in a week or month. The frequency is very important to document as that can determine whether your treatment should focus on an acute medication when you have an attack, or whether you need a preventive medication.

Talking About How You Manage Pain and Other Health Issues

> Doctors understand that patients try various over-the-counter and alternative treatments on their own, but many patients are either embarrassed to admit it to their doctors, or they don't realize that all treatments need to be discussed.

Over the years, I have had many patients not tell me about seeing chiropractors, acupuncturists, or any healthcare providers outside of traditional Western medicine. Sometimes, they admit to being afraid that I may not agree with what they were doing. Other times, they simply forgot to tell me, not thinking it was important to mention. But as a primary care physician and headache specialist, it is critically important for me to know about all the treatments or medications a patient is trying, including any over-the-counter products and treatments for unrelated conditions. Are you in so much pain that you are taking 6–12 Excedrin (acetaminophen-aspirin-caffeine) a day? You might be having rebound headache, which often comes from overuse of over-the-counter analgesic medicine.

If your doctor knows your current and past treatment regimen at the beginning of the visit, you can develop a successful headache treatment plan more quickly. For instance, if you are suffering from medication overuse headache, the focus of the visit needs to be on strategies to get out of rebound, including how to eliminate or taper down on the medication being overused.

Your doctor needs to know if you are using of these treatments:

- Over-the-counter pain relievers
- Prescription and over-the-counter medicines for allergies, cold and congestion symptoms, high blood pressure, depression, anxiety, bipolar disorder, or other medical conditions
- Supplements and vitamins
- Complementary and alternative treatments, such as acupuncture, biofeedback, physical therapy, and massage therapy
- Chiropractic treatment
- Oral contraceptives or other hormonal treatment

Taking Control

By now, you've realized that to feel better, you have to take an active role in the treatment and management of your headache condition. I recommend that you use your computer to keep a list of all current healthcare providers (include contact information); current medications (include dosage and how it is taken, for example twice a day); current daily supplements, such as vitamins and calcium; over-the-counter medications, whether taken daily or as needed such as Excedrin, Advil (ibuprofen), aspirin, or Tylenol (acetaminophen) (include frequency); and note any allergies. You may also consider listing medical conditions, past surgeries, past trauma, and family history. Past trauma should include head or neck injuries, because this history can be very important in evaluating headaches. This list should be updated as medications and information changes, and it can be printed out and brought to all your visits. Medical offices do keep their own history files but I still recommend you keep this list. It can be a good reference for you, your family, and all your treating providers. You should probably also keep a copy of it in your purse and another copy with a family member.

You may prefer to separate the medication list into medication taken for headaches versus medication taken for other medical conditions. Make sure to always include birth control pills or hormone products in your lists, including the name of the birth control pill. There are many generic versions available, and it is not always easy to identify a name brand. I recommend writing down the dose of the estrogen and progesterone on the medication list, or bring in the birth control pack with you for your visit. The dose of estrogen is often written as "ethinyl estradiol" (abbreviated as EE), and the usual dose ranges from 20 to 35 micrograms (mcg); it is the most common synthetic estrogen preparation in birth control pills. There are many different progesterone preparations in birth control pills, but that dose is not as critical to most headache providers because progesterone has not been as clearly linked to menstrual migraine as estrogen has. However, I like to know if a woman with menstrual migraine is on a monophasic or triphasic birth control pill. Monophasic means that all the "active" pills have the same amount of estrogen and progesterone, and this is usually reflected by all the active pills looking alike and being the same color in the pill pack. Monophasic pills are generally better tolerated in women with migraine and/or mood disorders. A triphasic birth control pill has fluctuating (changing) amounts of estrogen and/or progesterone in the pill pack. Typically, the color of the birth control pill changes to reflect the change in dose. These changing hormone levels can aggravate migraine and/or mood changes in a woman. Birth control pills can worsen *or* help migraine in women; it is often very helpful to know the dose of estrogen and progesterone in a woman's pill and where in the pill pack most of the migraines are occurring. A change in the birth control pill can sometimes make a huge improvement in migraine control for a woman.

Box 11-1

Nancy, the 29-year-old attorney we have been following, was frustrated with her family medicine physician, who did not have any new ideas for her disabling migraines and who referred Nancy to a local neurologist. Nancy made an appointment. The waiting room was filled with information on multiple sclerosis, stroke, seizures, and dementia. There were no brochures about headache. The neurologist ordered a magnetic resonance imaging (MRI) brain scan to make sure Nancy does not have a brain tumor. The MRI scan came out negative (normal). Nancy was reassured, but then wondered, "Now what?" The neurologist suggested Elavil (amitriptyline) for prevention. Nancy began taking the Elavil but began having side effects, including constipation and dry mouth. She did some research on the Internet and found that Elavil can also cause weight gain. Discouraged, she stopped the Elavil and asked the neurologist

(continued)

> **BOX 11-1 (Continued)**
>
> for other options. He suggested Inderal (propanolol) but Nancy was concerned because her blood pressure was already on the low side, and she read that Inderal can lower blood pressure as well as cause sedation (tiredness) and depression. She asked if there were other options, including a hormonal approach to her migraines. The neurologist replied, "I don't do anything with hormones. I am a neurologist, not a gynecologist. You need to ask your gynecologist about hormones." Nancy left the neurologist's office frustrated. She wondered if there was such a thing as a headache specialist.

Finding a Headache Specialist

A headache specialist can be a neurologist, family medicine provider, internist, dentist, psychologist, psychiatrist, nurse practitioner (NP), physician assistant (PA), or any healthcare provider who has a special interest and focus in treating the headache patient. To find a headache-focused provider in your area, go to one of several headache provider websites if your current treating providers are not aware of any offices in your area. In addition, these websites have a lot of educational information about headaches, and many have downloadable headache diaries (calendars) that can be printed out. The following are websites I recommend:

- www.headaches.org. Website for the National Headache Foundation (NHF)
- www.achenet.org. Website for the American Headache Society (AHS) Committee on Headache Education
- www.helpforheadaches.com. Website created and managed by Teri Robert, writer and patient advocate for headache sufferers

All of these websites have listings of headache-focused providers and clinics. For complete address and contact information for these websites, see the Appendix.

Most healthcare providers who are passionate about treating headache patients will be a member of the NHF, the AHS, or both. Both organizations offer educational programs for providers to learn about headache and to keep up with new treatments. To find out if a provider has a strong interest in headache, it may be worth asking if he or she is a member of these national organizations. Some headache providers may even be a member of the International Headache Society and attend headache conferences all over the world. In other cases, a provider may be a member of a regional headache organization, such as the Headache Cooperative of New England (HCNE) or the Headache Cooperative of the Pacific (HCOP). As a member of AHS, NHF, and HCOP, I credit these organizations and the educational programs they organize with helping me to keep up with the field of headache medicine.

There is an additional certification in headache that you can use to help identify headache specialists. The certification is through the United Council of Neurologic Subspecialties (UCNS). If you can find a physician with this certification, you can be assured a level of knowledge and experience in headache care that will benefit your treatment. To learn more about this certification, go to www. ucns.org.

Today, many headache fellowship programs are available in the United States, so some headache providers may have completed a headache fellowship after their medical residency program. Typically, headache fellowships are offered to neurology residents who have an interest in headache. Occasionally, a headache fellowship may be offered to a non-neurologist provider, such as an orofacial pain resident or internal medicine resident.

In some communities, headache clinics are especially designed to evaluate and treat challenging cases. Many of these are affiliated with university and teaching hospitals. Some of the better known include:

1. Jefferson Headache Center
   Thomas Jefferson University Hospital
   Philadelphia, Pennsylvania

2. Montefiore Headache Center
   Albert Einstein College of Medicine
   Bronx, New York

3. The Johns Hopkins Headache Center
   Johns Hopkins University
   Baltimore, Maryland

4. Dartmouth Headache Center
   Dartmouth Hitchcock Medical Center
   Lebanon, New Hampshire

5. Headache Center (Neurology Department)
   David Geffen School of Medicine
   University of Los Angeles (UCLA)
   Los Angeles, California

6. Headache Center (Neurology Department)
   University of Washington Medical Center
   Seattle, Washington

7. Headache Center (Neurology Department)
   Cleveland Clinic
   Cleveland, Ohio

8. Headache Center (Department of Neurology)
   University of San Francisco
   San Francisco, California

9. Mayo Clinic College of Medicine
   Rochester, Minnesota; Scottsdale, Arizona

10. University of Pittsburgh Headache Center
    Pittsburgh, Pennsylvania

11. Headache Center (Department of Neurology)
    University of Alabama
    Birmingham, Alabama

12. Stanford Headache Program
    Stanford University School of Medicine
    Stanford, California

There are also well-established headache centers such as the Diamond Headache Clinic in Chicago, Illinois, founded by Dr. Seymour Diamond. The Diamond Headache Clinic was the first headache-focused center established in the United States. Other well-known headache centers include:

- Michigan Head Pain and Neurological Institute, Ann Arbor, Michigan
- John Graham Headache Center, Boston, Massachusetts
- Cedars Sinai-The Headache & Pain Center, Cedars Sinai Medical Center, Los Angeles, California
- The Headache Center of Southern California, Encinitas, California
- Headache Care Center, Springfield, Missouri
- Anodyne Headache and PainCare, Dallas, Texas
- Houston Headache Clinic, Houston, Texas
- The Headache Institute, St. Luke's-Roosevelt Hospital, New York, New York
- Headache Center, Park Nicollet Health Services, Minneapolis, Minnesota
- New England Center for Headache, Stamford, Connecticut
- Hoag Headache and Facial Pain Program, Newport Beach, California

The Team Approach

At the newly formed Hoag Hospital Headache and Facial Pain Program, where I am one of the directors, we offer a multidisciplinary team approach for the management of headache and facial pain conditions. Psychiatrists, psychologists, pain specialists (including orofacial pain specialists), nurse navigators, in-hospital nurses, physical therapists, and headache-focused physicians meet regularly to discuss cases. A monthly support group for headache patients, community educational programs, and headache classes are all part of our program. Being part of this team approach allows me to better manage my headache patients, compared to being by myself in a solo medical practice, and I feel I have much more to offer my headache patients.

I encourage you to look for this type of team approach in the evaluation and treatment of your headaches if you are frustrated with your current headache management.

For a more complete listing of headache centers and clinics, go to www.achenet.org, www.headaches.org, or www.helpforheadaches.com.

What to Look for in a Headache Center

In my opinion, a good headache center should include not only expertise in evaluating your headache but should provide good communication with your other healthcare clinicians. Most of the time, you can be referred back to your primary care provider once you have been evaluated and put on a successful treatment plan by the specialty headache center. It is not necessary for most headache patients to continue to travel to specialty headache centers for their ongoing management. Ideally, a comprehensive consult report should be sent to your primary care provider, with a copy to for you, to support appropriate follow-up care.

In my practice, the office is electronic, and we can fax or e-mail the consult report to the patient's primary care provider. I can also print out my report and give it to a patient at the conclusion of the visit. Having a printed report can be very helpful in reinforcing our treatment plan. Be assertive and ask any provider evaluating your headaches to provide you with a copy of his of her report, for your review and files. It can be hard to remember everything that is discussed during an office visit; having a print-out to refer to can be very helpful.

> **BOX 11-2**
>
> Take charge of your medical care for your headaches. If the current treating providers you are seeing are not giving you the help that you feel you need, seek out a headache-focused specialist or headache center in your area. Your life is worth it! Don't sell yourself short when it comes to getting the help you need. See the Appendix for additional information regarding headache resources.

12

Conclusion

T HIS BOOK PROJECT HAS BEEN A 3-YEAR EFFORT, ONE characterized by episodic times of intense writing alternating with weeks of being put aside as my medical practice and "life" got in the way. As I re-read and edit the chapters, I am never 100% satisfied. New advances are being made in the headache field; new medications are being submitted for U.S. Food and Drug Administration (FDA) approval; and new insights into the genetics and cause of migraine are being discovered. As a result, some of the information printed in this book may not be completely up to date by the time of publication. At the end of the day, I settle for imperfection; otherwise, this book will never be published.

You will be the ultimate judge of whether the material in this book is helpful for you. Helping to lessen the burden of headache, including menstrual migraine, is a major passion for me, both in my medical practice and as I lecture on the subject to medical professionals. I have written many articles in medical journals and chapters on headache for medical textbooks. However, this book is my first attempt to reach out directly to migraine sufferers in a book. As I stated in the introduction, there are many books on the subject of headache for the lay public. There are also many books on the subject of women, menopause, and hormonal therapy. But there are few that cover both headache and hormones in women. I have tried to bridge that gap here and focus on women, hormones, and headache. Have I been successful? I welcome your feedback and suggestions. My e-mail is drhutchinson@ocmigraine.org.

I have attempted to make this subject of women and headaches both practical and approachable as I developed the characters of Beth, Lisa, Nancy, Melanie, Theresa, Christy, and Kate. Perhaps you have seen yourself in one or more of these women. Perhaps some of the treatment approaches have been helpful for you as you learn to manage your own disabling headaches and work with your physician and other healthcare providers.

Published research into the cause and treatment of migraine is increasing at a rapid rate. I encourage you to keep up with all that is happening in the headache world. One way to stay connected with the ever-evolving world of headache research, including menstrual migraine, is to get acquainted with several headache-focused websites and organizations. See the Appendix for a list of headache-related websites that I recommend.

In closing, I wish success for each of you. May your migraines, including menstrual migraines, be a minor inconvenience for you as you enjoy the life you were meant to live. Never give up on finding effective relief for your headaches, and never give up on yourself.

❖

Appendix
International Headache
Classification criteria

Tension-Type Headache Criteria

A. Individual must have had at least 10 episodes fulfilling criteria B–D

B. Headache lasts from 30 minutes to 7 days

C. Headache has two or more of the following characteristics:
   1. Bilateral location
   2. Pressing/tightening (nonpulsating) quality
   3. Mild or moderate intensity
   4. Not aggravated by routine physical activity

D. Both of the following:
   1. No nausea or vomiting
   2. No more than one of photophobia or phonophobia *(Note: photophobia refers to sensitivity to light; phonophobia refers to sensitivity to noise.)*

E. Cannot be attributed to another disorder

Tension headache may coexist with migraine. When it does, it tends to be more frequent and lasts longer in migraine sufferers than in nonmigraine individuals.

> *Note: Notice the description of mild-moderate in severity. If a headache is severe, it is most likely not tension headache. Also notice the lack of nausea and vomiting in the criteria.*

Cluster Headache Criteria

A. At least 5 attacks fulfilling criteria B–E

B. Severe or very severe unilateral orbital (one-sided in the eye area), supraorbital, and/or temporal pain lasting 15–180 minutes if untreated

C. Headache is accompanied by at least one of the following:
   1. Ipsilateral conjunctival injection and/or lacrimation
   2. Ipsilateral nasal congestion and/or rhinorrhea
   3. Ipsilateral eyelid edema
   4. Ipsilateral forehead and facial sweating
   5. Ipsilateral miosis and ptosis
   6. A sense of restlessness or agitation

D. Attacks have a frequency from one every other day to eight per day

E. They cannot be attributed to another disorder

> *Note: Unilateral refers to one-sided; orbital refers to the eye area; ipsilateral means "same side." In the case of cluster headache, this means that the associated symptoms, such as the eye being inflamed and tearing, occur on the same side as the headache. Cluster headache only occurs on one side of the head, unlike tension and migraine headaches, which are often on both sides of the head.*

Cluster headache is separated into two categories:

1. Episodic: Occurs in periods lasting 7 days to 1 year separated by pain-free periods lasting 1 month or more

2. Chronic: Attacks occur for more than 1 year without remission or with remission lasting less than 1 month

Note: Remission means the headache is not present.

Migraine Without Aura (Common Migraine) Criteria

A. At least five attacks fulfilling criteria B–D
B. Headache attacks lasting 4–72 hours (untreated or unsuccessfully treated)
C. Headache has at least two of the following characteristics:
1. Unilateral location (one sided)
2. Pulsating quality
3. Moderate or severe pain intensity
4. Aggravation by or causing avoidance of routine physical activity (e.g., walking or climbing stairs)
D. During headache, at least one of the following:
1. Nausea and/or vomiting
2. Photophobia (sensitivity to light) and phonophobia (sensitivity to sound)
E. Cannot be attributed to another disorder

According to these criteria, menstrual migraine is migraine without aura that occurs within 2 days of the onset of menstruation to 3 days after. Menstrual migraine is separated into two categories:

1. *Pure menstrual migraine*: Migraine attacks occur only in relationship to menstruation. Specifically, attacks occur within the 2 days prior to 3 days after menstruation. To meet the criteria, a woman must experience these migraine attacks in at least two out of every three cycles or 66% of the time.
2. *Menstrual-related migraine*: Migraine attacks that occur in at least two out of three cycles within the time frame of 2 days prior and 3 days after menstruation. Migraine attacks occur at other times of the month as well.

The majority of women with menstrual migraine are categorized as having menstrual-related migraine, as opposed to pure menstrual migraine. Most women with menstrual migraine have migraines from other triggers at other times in their cycle. Other common triggers include stress, lack of sleep, skipped meals, food additives, preservatives, and changes in barometric pressure.

Migraine with Aura (Classic Migraine) Criteria

A. At least two attacks fulfilling criteria B–D

B. Aura consisting of at least one of the following, but no motor weakness:
   1. Fully reversible visual symptoms including positive features (e.g., flickering lights, spots, or lines) and/or negative features (i.e., loss of vision)
   2. Fully reversible sensory symptoms including positive features (i.e., pins and needles) and/or negative features (i.e., numbness)
   3. Fully reversible dysphasic speech disturbance

C. At least two of the following:
   1. Homonymous visual symptoms and/or unilateral sensory symptoms
   2. At least one aura symptom develops gradually over 5 or more minutes and/or different aura symptoms occur in succession over 5 or more minutes
   3. Each symptom lasts for 5 or more minutes and less than 60 minutes

D. Headache fulfilling criteria B–D for migraine without aura begins during the aura or follows the aura within 60 minutes

E. Cannot be attributed to another disorder

Headache Resources & Organizations

1. American Headache Society Committee on Headache Education www.achnet.org
Educational website sponsored by the American Headache Society, a professional society dedicated to the study of headache and facial pain.

2. National Headache Foundation (NHF)
www.headaches.org
Educational website offered by The National Headache Foundation, a non-profit organization dedicated to providing education about headache to professionals and patients; publishes a monthly e-newsletter; publishes a magazine Head Wise Magazine; membership is $20/year for patients

3. www.helpforheadaches.com
Website of Teri Robert, writer and patient advocate for headache
Filled with valuable information for headache patients

4. www.headachecare.com
Website for the nationally accredited Headache Care Center in Springfield, Missouri
Contains educational materials to help the headache patient including the ability to order a home biofeedback kit

5. www. Migraine.com
Interactive headache-focused website for migraine headache sufferers
Includes blog for Dr. Hutchinson and expert opinion articles

6. www.MyMigraineConnection.com
Educational information about migraines (part of HealthCentral)

7. www.mychronicmigraine.com

Information focused on those having headache 15 or more days a month

8. www.iHeadacheApp.com

Instructions on how to install this app for electronic devices; tracks headaches including frequency, type of headache, medication usage and disability scale; eliminates the hassle of keeping paper diary; is free for most electronic devices

Recommended Reading

1. The Keeler Migraine Method: A Groundbreaking, Individualized Treatment Program from the Renowned Headache Clinic. Written by: Robert Cowan, MD

2. The Woman's Migraine Toolkit: Managing Your Headaches from Puberty to Menopause. Written by: Dawn Marcus, MD and Philip Bain, MD

3. Conquering Your Migraine. Written by: Seymour Diamond, MD, with Mary A. Franklin.

4. Living Well with Migraine Disease & Headaches. Written by: Teri Robert, Patient Advocate.

5. Chocolate & Vicodin Written by: Jennette Fulda (headache sufferer)

Breastfeeding Resources

Medications and Mothers' Milk 2010 Fourteenth Edition
Thomas Hale, PhD
To order online, go to http://www.ibreastfeeding.com
Considered the most authoritative and up-to-date resource on the use of medications in breastfeeding mothers; good reference for all health care professionals who work with breastfeeding mothers and babies

Mini Medications and Mothers' Milk 2010 Fourteenth Edition

Thomas Hale, PhD

Smaller, more concise version

Same online ordering information

Recommended for any woman concerned about medication use, including migraine medication, during breastfeeding

On-line Data Base for medications & breast-feeding

National Institutes of Health

To access: toxnet.nlm.nih.gov/cgi-bin/sis/htmlgen?LACT

Enter name of medication and information from available studies is shown helping to make a decision about whether to take a medication if breast-feeding

Free service; no password needed

Index